CHARGE YOUR FOOD,

CHANGE YOUR LIFE

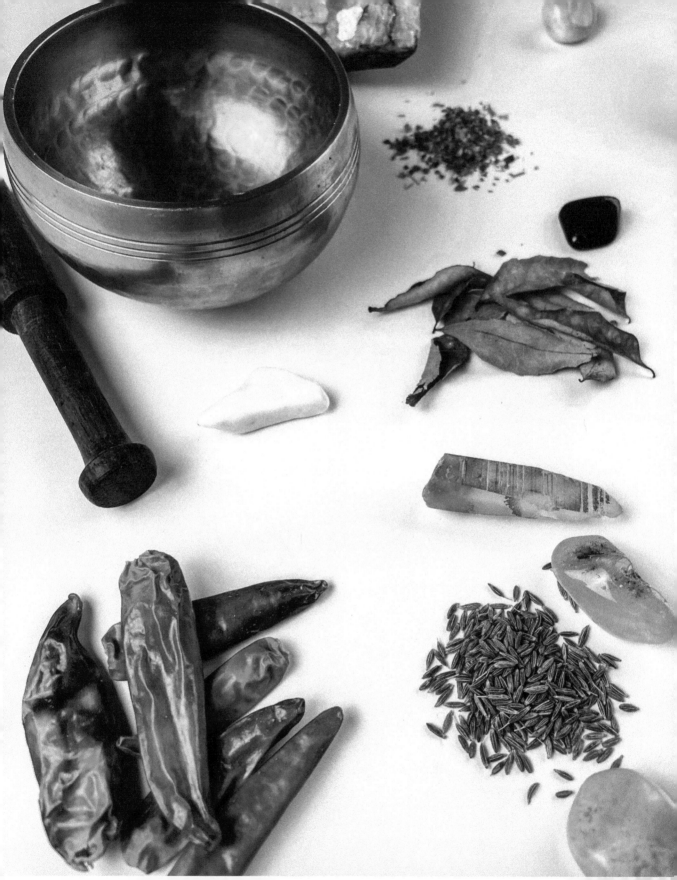

CHARGE YOUR FOOD, CHANGE YOUR LIFE

A Reiki Cookbook

CHRISTINA MANNING & JESSICA DUNAGAN

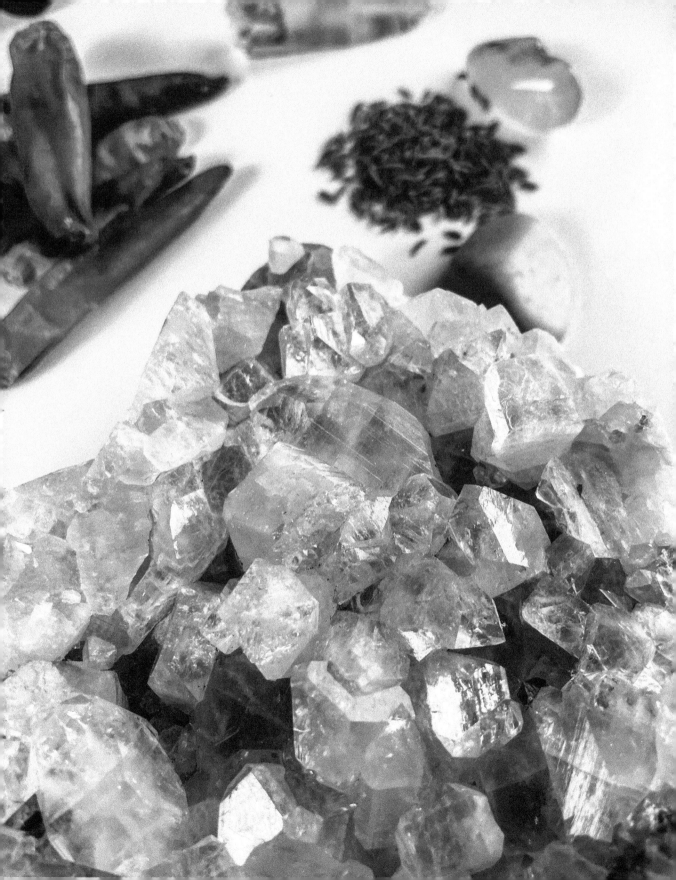

Dedicated

to the

most magical

never-to-be-tamed

provokingly adventurous little souls

whom we call

our children

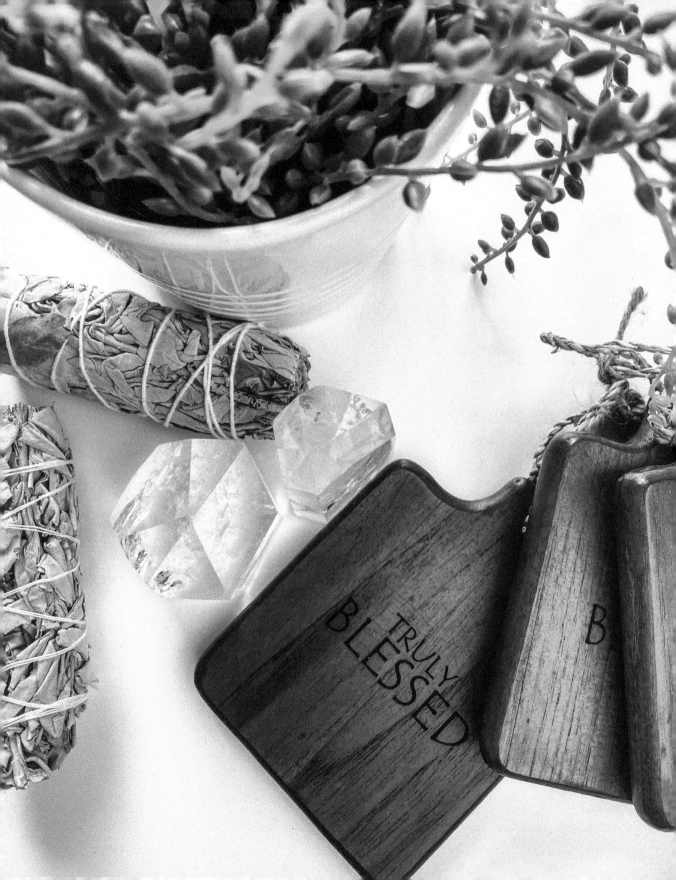

CONTENTS

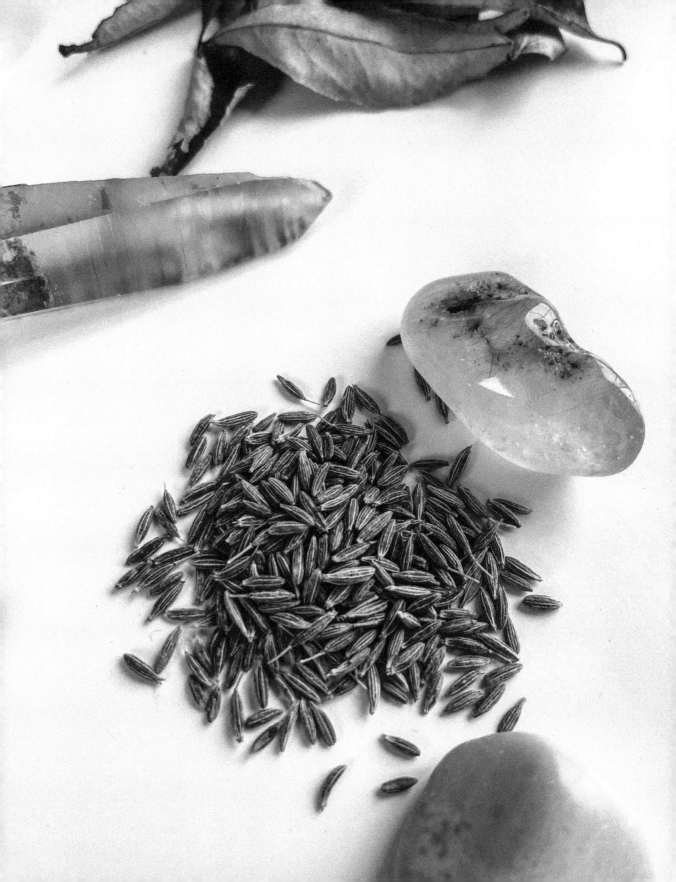

INTRODUCTION

Wow, we are so excited to share with you a new revolutionary way to cook your food! Not only is this book filled with recipes that we prepare for our family and grew up on, but we are going to teach you how to reiki charge your food! Do not feel overwhelmed, I know a lot of you are unaware of what Reiki even is, but that is why we will guide you through it. We will introduce you to what Reiki is, how to charge your food, and give you affirmations before you even use our recipes.

But first, who are we? Why did we write this book? And what led us to reiki charging our food?

Who are we? We are Christina and Jessica, and we are identical twin sisters. We grew up on a farm in Oregon and we ate fresh ingredients from the garden. Our Mother did not have a lot of money and so she made our dinner with minimal ingredients. Some of these recipes we share in this book such as her zucchini bread and chicken noodle soup. After we left home, we started to do what most young adults do, we ate fast food and takeout – contaminating our bodies with toxins, processed foods, and refined carbs. Around this same time, our lives unexpectedly changed. We both became suddenly ill and gained over 100 pounds combined. At the time, we were naïve and did not realize how the foods we were eating were not helping to assist our bodies in dealing with our health issues. The doctors finally diagnosed us with Hyperinsulinemia – a rare genetic disease that made our bodies over produce insulin. Eating processed foods, and high sugar content, were hurting us more than helping us. We also became hyper focused on negative thoughts, telling ourselves, "we are sick", "we are fat", "we will never feel healthy again."

One afternoon we realized that what we were doing was not working. We were only getting worse, gaining more weight, and feeling less hopeful about a positive outcome. That is when we were guided to learn about Reiki and the power of our mind and thoughts. The energy was more powerful than we had realized. That is when we went on a personal quest to heal our health issues using Reiki energy. Do not worry if you are a beginner with Reiki, in this book we will share with you what reiki is, and how you can use it to charge your food.

We started using reiki energy to charge our food and we used the power of our energy to start to create a new path for our life. We charged every meal we ate and started to notice that we were feeling better, we were losing the weight, and we were beginning to see results. We also started choosing healthier foods that assisted in healing our bodies, and we will share those recipes in this book.

So, why did we write this book? We wrote this book because we want to share our success with you and help awaken others. This is such a powerful gift that each one of us have and we hope that it will help change the way we eat our food. It is so fun to reiki charge our food and use that energy to help manifest our lives. They say, we are what we eat, so why not eat food that has been charged with your intentions and manifestations. Let this book be a personal guide for you. Explore what Reiki is, and how to charge your food. After that, look through our intention pages and find an intention that you would like to charge your food with. Follow that up by finding a recipe that you want to try. Lastly, enjoy your meal and watch your life change. Charge your food and change your life! Many blessings from our table to yours!

WHAT IS REIKI? Reiki energy is a form of energy healing that was discovered in Japan during the late 1800's. Our entire bodies are made up of energy and we carry an unseen "life force" of energy that flows through us. Reiki is used to administer that energy we harbor and pass it on to others or objects by the "laying of hands". When used on others it can promote healing and relaxation, but when used on objects it can transfer your intentions of energy into the object.

No one needs to be intimidated by reiki no matter what your skill level is. Reiki is a natural method of spiritual healing and self-improvement that everyone can use. Reiki energy is simple, you pass your energy through your hands.

The ability to learn Reiki is not dependent on intellectual capacity, nor do you have to be able to meditate. It also does not take years to master or learn. It is simply the transfer of energy. Many people hear reiki and assume that they have to have it done on them from a teacher or master of reiki but that is not the case, it is a form of healing that we can do on ourselves and to others by simply knowing how to do it. In this book, we will show you how to do reiki, how to manifest, and then how to charge your food.

Reiki is a pure form of healing and the best way to start using reiki to your advantage is to start learning how to channel the energy within you. The best way to do this is to start with a meditation to harbor the energy within you.

Here is a great exercise to try: Start by grounding yourself and getting comfortable in a calming environment. This can be a place to sit or rest, but it needs to be quiet and without distractions. Imagine there are roots extending from your seat and feet and moving down into the earth. This is the best way to feel like you are grounded. Once you feel rooted, imagine a white light of energy coming down from the universe and into the top of your head. Move this light of energy down throughout your body as it travels to your feet. Inhale this light as you feel it coming in with every breath. Exhale any pain, fear or negativity. You can imagine that what you exhale is grey. Continue to inhale the white light of the universe and fill your body up with it and exhale the grey. Continue to do this for as long as you desire until you are completely relaxed.

Now that you have learned what reiki is and how to charge yourself with the, "unseen lifeforce" you can move on to learn about manifesting. By combining the art of reiki with the power of manifesting, you will be charging your food before you know it!

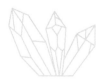

WHAT IS MANIFESTATION? To begin, I am sure you have heard of the word, "manifest" or "law of attraction", as it has been a popular trend these days. In a nutshell, manifestation is the idea that you bring something into your life through attraction and believe, i.e. if you think it, it will come. Our thoughts are energy and what we think, we become. Creating the life that you want is easy if you know how to use energy to attract what you belief you can achieve and deserve.

To start manifesting you must first be truly clear and concise on your goals. Manifesting can be approached differently by each person, but we do believe that manifesting is simple by following the same basic principles. First, you need to know what you want. It is easy to confuse the universe when you are unsure of what you want. It is so important to have a clear picture of what you want and where you see yourself going in your life.

Second, you need to ask the universe for what you want. This can be done with a vision board and/or writing a list of your intentions. Speaking your intentions out loud to the universe is another way to ask for what you want. Asking for what you want is simply creating an energetic force to create a space where you are putting out the "feelings" associated with the desire to have this item or goal. What energy we put out to the universe is being sent back to us and we are living that in our reality. For example, have you noticed that when you are thinking negative and focusing on your bad day that your feelings you project are negative? It seems like those "bad" days tend to stay bad or get worse as the day continues. That is the idea and principle that you are manifesting more negative experiences by projecting that energy and those feelings.

Lastly, you want to be grateful and to "receive" the gifts you manifest from the universe. While you may not get everything you envision in the order and the time frame you want, you should receive and acknowledge what you do get. It is especially important that you "act as if". A part of receiving what you manifest is to act as if it is already there. For example, say thank you to the universe for giving you what you manifest. Also, make sure you keep a positive mindset and stay focused on your vision. It is important to remove any obstacles which may cloud your vision, including fear and negative self-talk. For example, if you frequently find yourself questioning your worth or saying, "I don't deserve this," then counteract that by thinking of all the reasons why you are deserving.

The best part about manifestation is that it has no limits. You do not have to think small; it is ok to be a dreamer. The law of attraction knows no bounds. "Once you start dialing in your manifestation process, there's no limit to what—or how often or much—you manifest." With this book we are going to teach you to how use the power of reiki and manifesting to charge your food.

HOW TO CHARGE YOUR FOOD. Now that you have the basics of what Reiki and manifesting is, we will show you how to incorporate these abilities to reiki charge your food.

The first thing you will want to do is to prepare the ingredients and gather the food items you will need for the recipe. We have over 75 recipes that you can prepare if that makes this process easier for you. We recommend that you set aside three ingredients that you would like to reiki charge. The largest food item and the liquid ingredients are usually the best candidates to reiki charge, as they have more mass and easier energy components to charge.

Next, you will want to plan an intention in which you want to manifest. We have included intentions in this book to help guide you with affirmations that you can utilize. It is important that you are clear and concise on what your intention is and what energy you are trying to charge into your food. For example, if you have an audition coming up and you would like to be successful at it, we recommend that you use the affirmations that attract confidence.

Once you have prepared your food items to charge, along with the intention you plan to manifest, you can begin the process to charge your food. What is so amazing about reiki, is that you can use your power of manifesting to put this energy into the food you are about to eat. It is a way to not only take this time to manifest your dream, but to also put that energy into the food you are about to put into your body. Our cells and DNA are such magical entities, and they are what keeps us alive. You are now changing the molecular shape of your food's energy to now ingest and put into the cells of your body.

So, let us begin:

Step 1. Set out the items you want to charge. (You will reiki charge each item individually)

Step 2. Close your eyes, rub your hands together, and visualize the goal that you are wanting to manifest.

Step 3. Open your eyes and place your hands over the item you would like to reiki charge.

Step 4. Speak the intentions out loud as you transfer that energy into the food with your hands. It is important that as you state your intention you feel the love and joy that you would get from receiving that manifestation.

Step 5. Once you are done charging your food you can cook your recipe as you desire.

Step 6. Once the recipe is prepared, place your hands over the finished meal and state your intentions out loud one last time.

Step 7. Be grateful for your meal by saying, "Thank you" to the universe for giving you the intention you are manifesting. Say Thank you and enjoy your meal!

CHOOSE AN INTENTION. Here is a list of a few intentions you can use to charge your food. Of course with anything you are Reiki charging, your own personal manifestations are key. But here is a list of ideas and intentions you can use.

Intention 1. I attract an abundance of love.

Intention 2. I attract the life I want.

Intention 3. I am a money magnet.

Intention 4. Positivity always surrounds me.

Intention 5. Love comes to me easily.

Intention 6. Money flows into my life easily.

Intention 7. I ace the test.

Intention 8. Laughter is always surrounding me.

Intention 9. My life is peaceful.

Intention 10. I am successful.

Intention 11. I am enough.

Intention 12. I am beautiful and confident.

Intention 13. I create happiness in all that I do.

Intention 14. Everyone loves to be around me and has faith in me.

Intention 15. I am honest and truthful with myself.

Intention 16. I create a safe and secure space for myself in my life.

Intention 17. I am confident.

Intention 18. I am sexy.

Intention 19. I allow myself space to grow.

Intention 20. I am intuitive and listen to my gut.

Intention 21. There is an abundance of joy all around me.

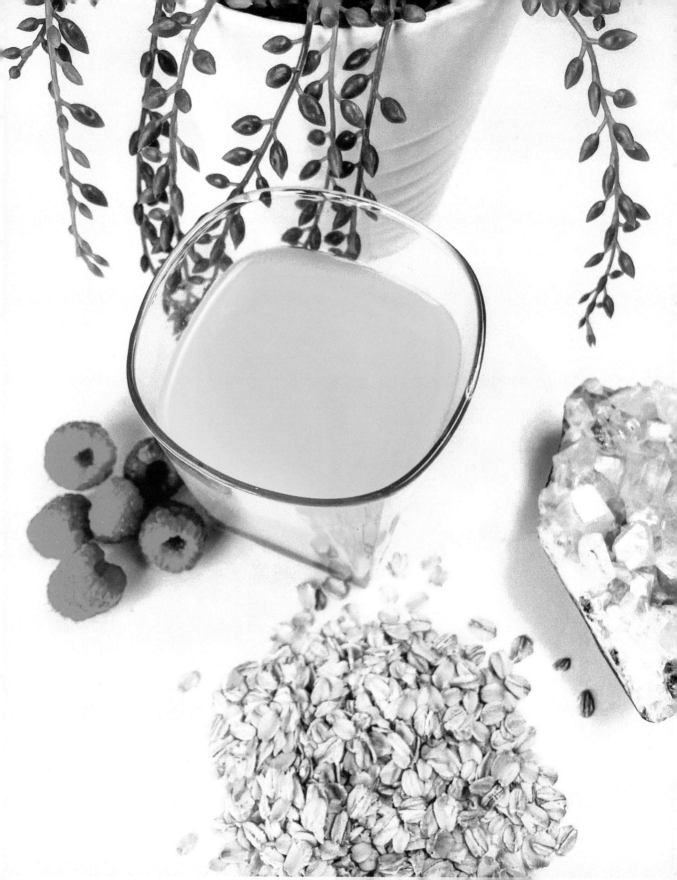

BREAKFASTS

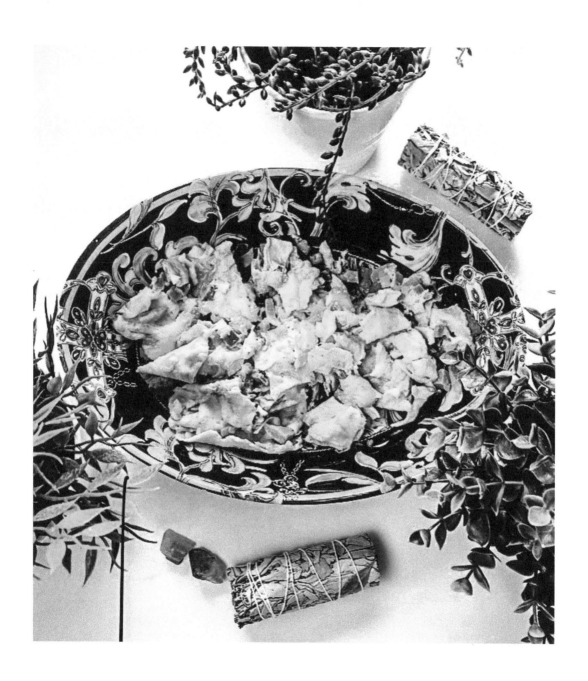

FARMER'S BREAKFAST SKILLET

½ lb bacon
1 20 oz package refrigerated diced
   potatoes
½ medium onion, diced
½ medium red bell pepper, diced
½ medium green bell pepper,
   diced
8 oz cubed ham
12 large eggs
½ cup half & half or heavy cream
1 cup shredded cheddar cheese
Seasoned salt and black pepper to
   taste

1. Preheat the oven to 350°F.

2. In an oven safe skillet, cook the bacon until crisp. Remove the bacon and keep the drippings in the pan.

3. Saute the bell peppers and onions in the remaining bacon grease over medium heat until soft.

4. Add the diced potatoes to the pan and cook for 6-8 minutes, stir until lightly browned and heated through.

5. Layer the potatoes evenly on the bottom of the skillet. Top the potatoes with the cubed ham. Top with ½ - of the shredded cheese

6. Whip the eggs with the half & half or cream. Season lightly with seasoned salt and black pepper. Pour on top.

7. Sprinkle with the remaining shredded cheese.

8. Place into the oven and bake for 15-20 minutes or until the eggs are fully cooked.

9. When finished baking, toss in a bowl with capers and freshly squeezed lemon juice from the lemon.

◇ OPTIONAL: Some people enjoy topping this breakfast skillet with country style gravy or hollandaise sauce before baking. (See dips & sauces for recipe)

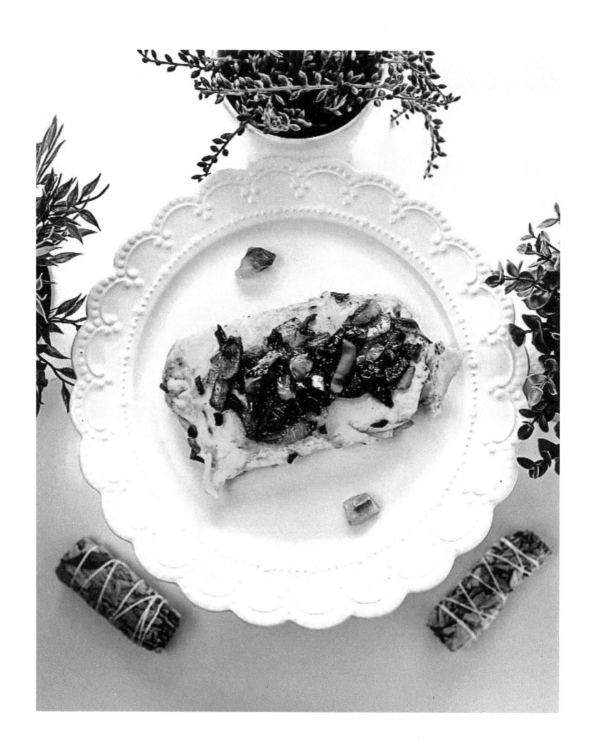

SOUTHWESTERN OMELETTE

½ lb ground turkey
½ medium onion, diced
½ medium red bell pepper, diced
½ medium green bell pepper,
   diced
½ medium tomato diced
1 packet of taco seasoning
6 large eggs
½ cup half & half or heavy cream
1 cup shredded cheddar cheese
Seasoned salt and black pepper to
   taste

1. In a stove top skillet, cook the ground turkey until fully browned. Follow the directions on the taco seasoning and add to the turkey. Set aside.

2. Saute the bell peppers and onions with a dash of olive oil until softened. Add to the taco seasoned turkey meat, stir over low- medium heat. Remove from heat and set aside.

3. Whip the eggs with the half & half or cream. Season lightly with seasoned salt and black pepper.

4. In a new skillet, add a dash of olive oil. Add the whipped eggs into the skillet over medium-low heat. Allow the eggs to cook entirely at the bottom of the pan without touching them or scrambling them.

5. Once the eggs appear cooked, add the taco meat that you set aside. Layer with ½ cup of shredded cheese.

6. With a spatula lightly fold over the eggs to form an omelette.

7. Top with the remaining shredded cheese and diced tomatoes.

_____

◊ OPTIONAL: Add sour cream and/or sliced avocado for garnish

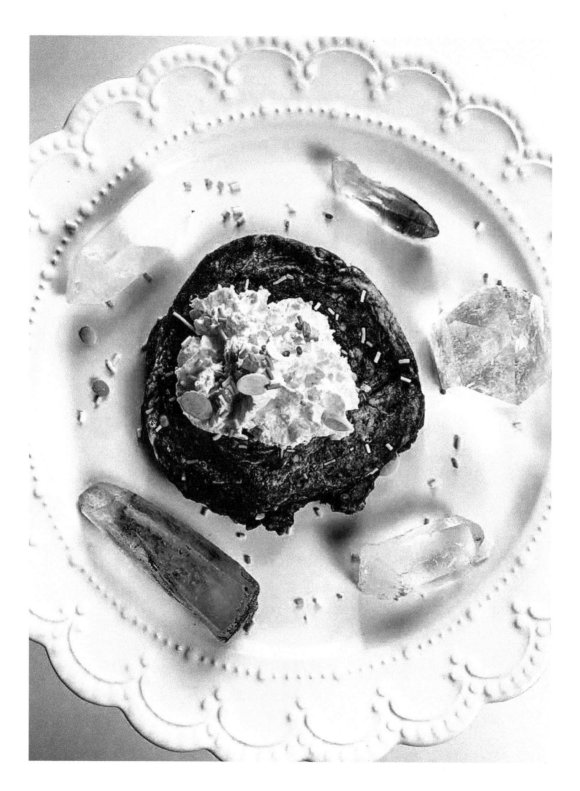

UNICORN PANCAKE

These pancakes are a super magical way to start your morning and the kids love it! It's perfect to pair these pancakes with positivity and excitement based intentions. We love to let the kids help in the kitchen and they find it so fun to reiki charge the sprinkles!

1½ cups all purpose flour
1¼ cups milk
3½ baking powder
1 large egg
1 tsp salt
1 tbsp sugar
3 tbsp melted butter
1 tbsp pastel colored sprinkles
¼ cup Nestle Unicorn chocolate chips

1. Prepare the kitchen with a large mixing bowl and a skillet on the stove.

2. In a large mixing bowl, sift together the flour, salt, & baking powder.

3. Stir in the remaining ingredients.

4. Heat a lightly oiled griddle or skillet over medium-high heat. Pour or scoop the batter onto the griddle, using approximately ¼ cup for each pancake. Brown on both sides and serve hot.

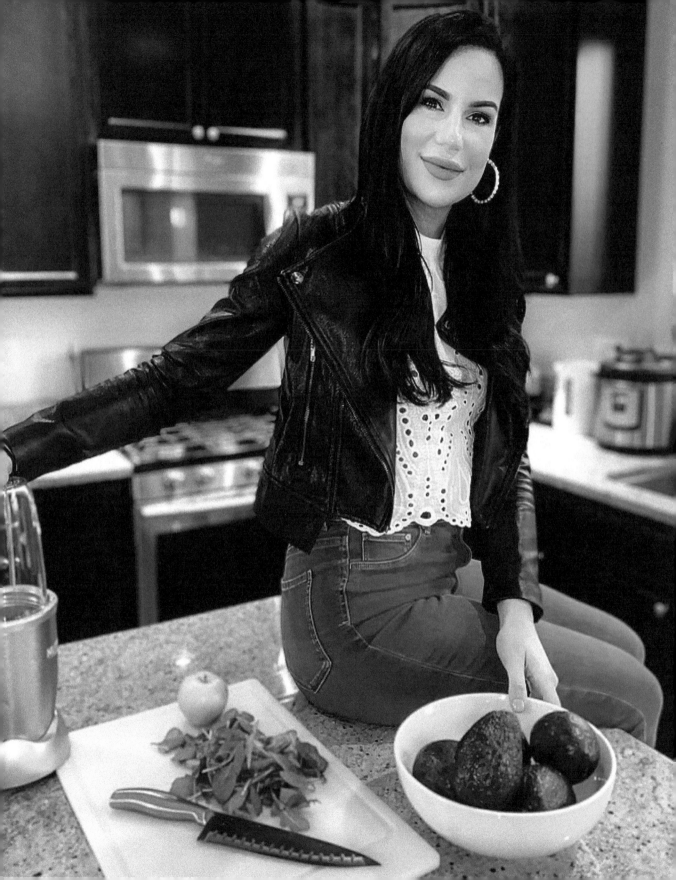

CHRISTINA'S GREEN POWER SMOOTHIE

Hi there, Christina here. I am so excited to share this recipe with you. Green smoothies are one of my favorite morning routines that I share with my kids. When my kids were little, I used to call these green smoothies, "Ice Cream" and they would light up with excitement. Nourishing my body is very important to me and so I love to include these smoothies packed with superfoods into my diet.

After suffering from a few health ailments, I researched how important our diets were in correlation with our health. I started a plant based diet and my health quickly improved and I felt the best I had ever felt. This was all the proof I needed.

What excites me the most about this, is that, not only am I nourishing my body, but I am also using reiki to charge the food and higher the energy vibration. I feel instantly happy, with a boost of energy.

1 ¼ cup unsweetened almond milk
½ cup frozen blueberries
½ cup raspberries
½ banana
½ cup spinach
½ cup kale
1 tbsp almond butter

1. In a blender of your choosing, prepare the settings for blend.

2. Place the spinach, kale, and almond milk into the blender. Blend until fully blended and the milk has turned completely green.

3. Add the rest of the ingredients.

4. Blend until smooth.

◊ OPTIONAL: 1 scoop of powdered greens or protein powder. 1 tsp of chia seeds or flax seeds.

HAM AND CHEESE SCRAMBLE

6 large eggs
1 tbsp of heavy cream
8 oz cubed ham
½ cup of shredded cheddar cheese
Seasoned salt and black pepper to
    taste

1. In a medium size bowl, whip eggs, heavy cream, and salt & pepper to taste.

2. Add the cubed ham to the bowl.

3. Heat a skillet on medium-low heat.

4. Add the eggs and ham. Scramble the eggs and ham until they are fluffy and fully cooked.

5. Top the scrambled eggs with shredded cheese and allow to melt.

EGGS BENEDICT

4 pieces of Canadian bacon
4 large eggs
2 tsp white or rice vinegar
2 English muffins
2 tbsp chopped parsley, for garnish

For Hollandaise sauce, see Dips &
   Sauces

1. Prepare the kitchen with a skillet and prepare the hollandaise sauce.

2. Heat a large skillet on medium-low heat. Add the Canadian bacon. Slowly fry, turning occasionally, until the bacon is browned on both sides.

3. Bring a large saucepan two-thirds filled with water to a boil, then add the vinegar. Bring the water to a boil again, then lower the heat to a bare simmer.

4. One egg at a time, crack an egg into a small bowl and slip it into the barely simmering water. Once it begins to solidify, you can slip in another egg, until you have all four cooked.

5. Toast the English muffins.

6. Assemble the dish. Place the Canadian bacon slice on the English muffin, followed by the poached egg. Top with hollandaise sauce and garnish with parsley.

FRENCH TOAST

6 slices of thick bread
   (Preferably potato bread)
2 large eggs
⅔ cup milk
¼ tsp of cinnamon
¼ tsp of nutmeg
1 tsp vanilla extract
1 tbsp butter, softened
½ cup strawberries, sliced

1. In a stove top skillet, melt a small slice of butter over low heat.

2. In a medium size bowl, beat together the eggs, milk, cinnamon, nutmeg, and vanilla extract.

3. Dip both sides of bread into the egg mixture, fully coating each side.

4. Turn the skillet to a medium- low heat.

5. Place the coated slice of bread into the skillet and cook on each side until golden brown.

◊ OPTIONAL: Coat each piece of french toast with butter, strawberries, and/or syrup and whipped cream.

PEANUT BUTTER BANANA SMOOTHIE

1 cup frozen yogurt
1 cup chocolate milk
2 tablespoons peanut butter
1 frozen banana

1. Place all ingredients in a blender and blend until smooth and creamy.

FRUIT BOWL WITH CHIA SEEDS

½ cup strawberries sliced
1 whole banana
½ cup raspberries
½ cup grapes
½ cup blueberries
2 tablespoons chia seeds

1. Wash and prepare your fruit.

2. Add to a bowl.

3. Top the fruit with chia seeds

BISCUITS & GRAVY

1 package of jumbo premade
   buttermilk biscuits
1 lb breakfast sausage, mild
⅓ cups all purpose flour
3 cups milk
Seasoned salt and black pepper to
   taste

1. Preheat your oven and follow the directions to bake the biscuits.

2. In a large skillet cook the sausage over medium-high heat until browned and fully cooked.

3. Reduce the heat to medium-low. Add milk and flour and stir thoroughly. Add the salt and pepper to taste. Stir occasionally until thickens. Typically 10-12 mins.

4. Spoon the gravy over warm biscuits and serve immediately while warm.

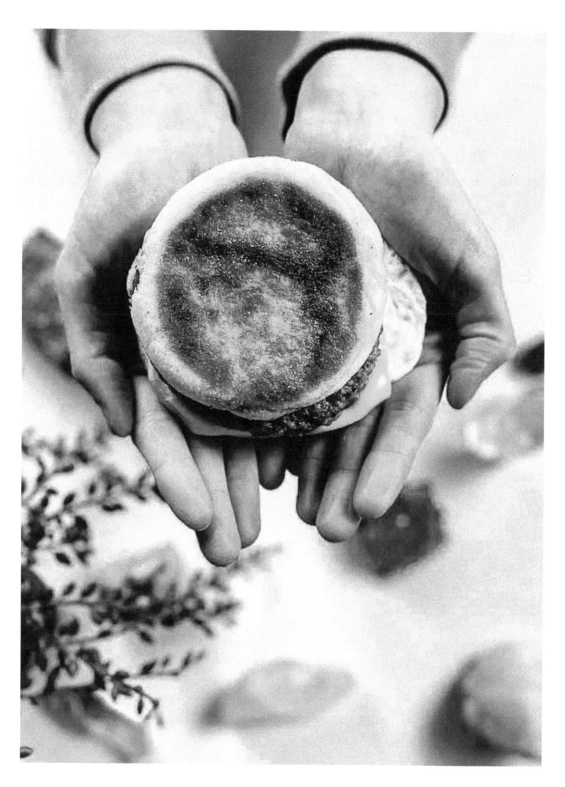

SAUSAGE AND EGG BREAKFAST SANDWICH

1 precooked sausage patty
1 egg
1 slice of American cheese
1 English muffin
1 tablespoon butter

1. Turn the stove burner on low-medium heat.

2. Add ½ tablespoon of butter until melted.

3. Crack the egg and cook on each side for 2 minutes.

4. Remove and set aside. (It should be cooked throughout unless you like a runny yolk).

5. Cook the precooked sausage patty on each side for 3 minutes. You want it to be cooked and heated through.

6. Add a slice of cheese and the egg on top of the patty. Keep it in the pan until the cheese is melted. Set aside.

7. Add ½ tablespoon of butter in the pan to melt. Coat the bottom sides of the English muffin and let them crisp. Add the patty and egg and brown the sandwich on each side.

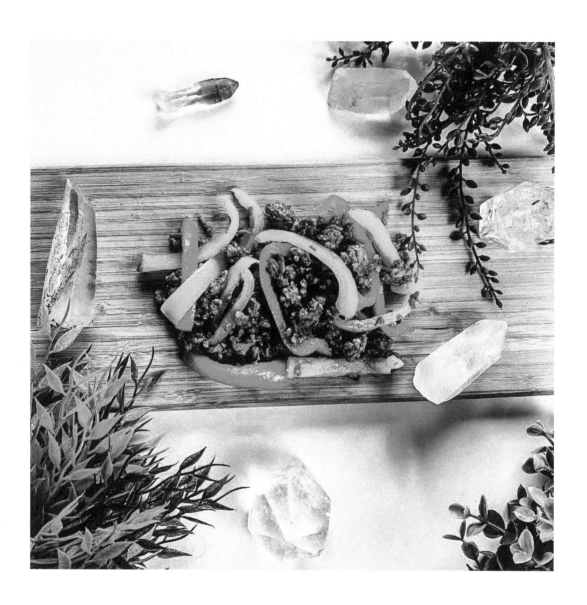

SAUSAGE AND PEPPER

¼ cup extra-virgin olive oil
1 lb of sweet italian sausage
2 red bell peppers, sliced
1 sweet yellow onion, sliced
1 teaspoon salt
1 teaspoon pepper
4 garlic cloves, chopped
4 to 6 hoagie rolls, optional

1. Heat the oil in a heavy large skillet over medium heat.

2. Add the sausage and cook until brown on both sides, about 7 to 10 minutes.

3. Remove the sausage from the pan and drain

4. Keep the pan over medium heat and add the peppers, onions, salt and pepper.

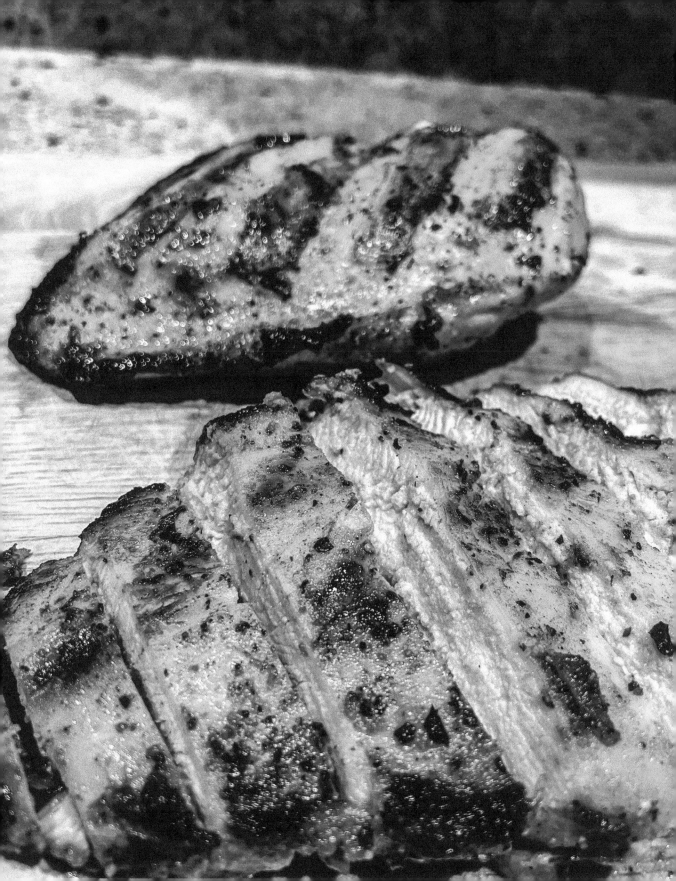

ENTREES

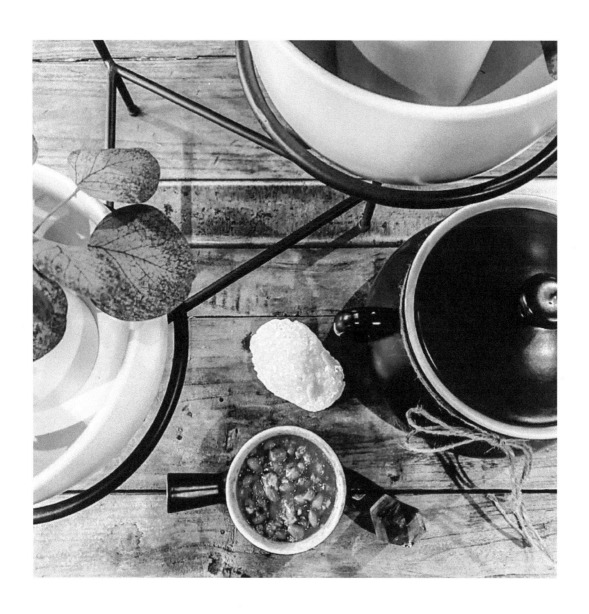

CHILI

½ lb italian sausage
½ lb ground beef
½ medium onion, diced
½ medium red bell pepper, diced
½ medium green bell pepper,
   diced
1 packet chili seasoning, only use
   2 tbsp of the powder.
1 tbsp brown sugar
¾ cup beef stock
¾ cup red wine
1 28 oz can of chopped tomatoes
1 15 oz can of kidney bean,
   drained
2 tbsp olive oil
Seasoned salt and black pepper to
   taste

1. In a large skillet, cook the sausage and beef until fully cooked.

2. To the same skillet, add the bell peppers, onions and season with salt and pepper until the vegetables are tender.

3. Over medium-high heat add the beef stock, wine, brown sugar, chili powder, and stir until it starts to boil.

4. Reduce the heat and add the tomatoes and beans.

5. Reduce the heat to medium-low and let it simmer for 2 hours.

6. Serve with toppings of choice.

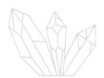

WHITE BEAN SOUP

1 large can of white great northern beans, drained
10 cups of vegetable stock
½ medium onion, diced
4 garlic cloves, minced
10 cherry tomatoes, halved
1 large carrot, sliced
2 celery stalks, sliced
½ tbsp rosemary, finely chopped
½ tbsp parsley, finely chopped
2 tbsp olive oil
Seasoned salt and black pepper to taste

1. In a large pot, heat olive oil on medium heat.

2. Add rosemary and garlic. Saute.

3. To the same pot, add carrots, celery, and onions. Saute until veggies are still crispy, not fully tender.

4. Add vegetable stock.

5. Bring the soup to a boil.

6. Once boiling, reduce heat and add the tomatoes and beans.

7. Simmer for 40 minutes.

8. Add the parsley and use some to garnish each bowl.

CAULIFLOWER RICE STIR FRY

2 tbsp coconut oil
1 package of frozen cauliflower
   rice
½ medium onion, diced
½ medium red bell pepper, diced
½ carrot, sliced
7 brussel sprouts, quartered
7 broccoli florets
1 tsp sesame oil
1 tbsp soy sauce
Seasoned salt and black pepper to
   taste

1. In a large skillet, melt the coconut oil on medium-high heat.

2. Add the onion, bell pepper, carrot, brussel sprouts, and broccoli and sautee until tender.

3. Add the defrosted cauliflower rice and stir while cooking.

4. Once fully cooked, stir in the sesame oil, soy sauce, and season with salt & pepper.

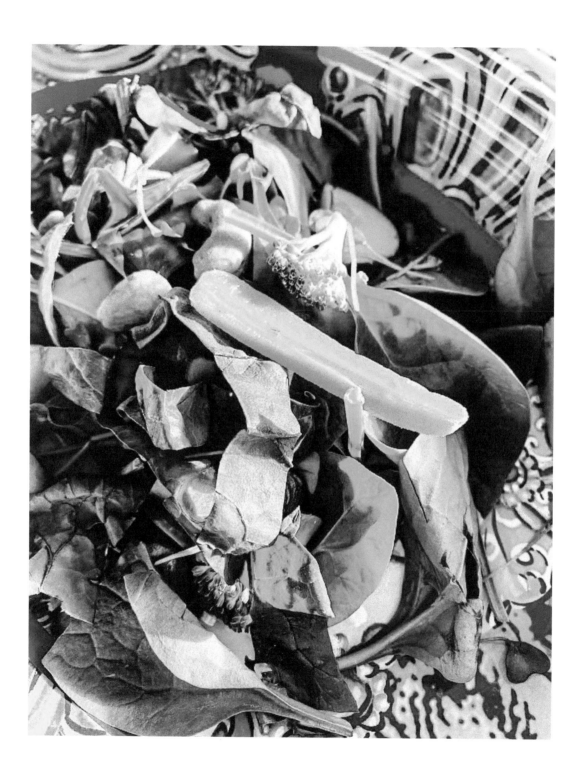

SUPERFOOD SALAD

1 cup baby spinach
1 cup chard, chopped
½ cup baby arugula
½ medium red bell pepper, diced
½ carrot, sliced
8 cherry tomatoes, halved
½ avocado, diced
¼ cup cashews
1 tbsp olive oil
Seasoned salt and black pepper to
  taste

1. In a large serving bowl, combine all ingredients.

2. Toss evenly.

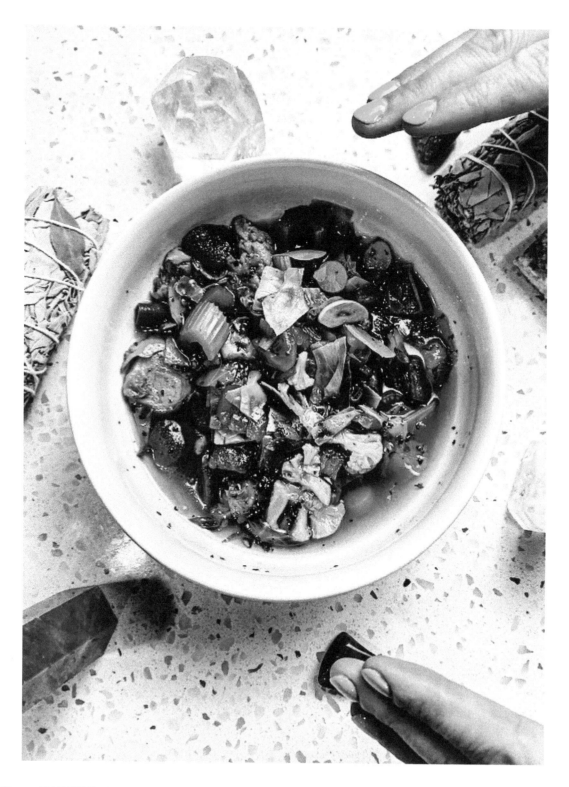

INSTANT POT VEGGIE SOUP

½ head of cabbage, finely diced
2 celery stalks, diced
½ medium onion, diced
1 large carrot, sliced
8 brussel sprouts, quartered
10 green beans, sliced
6 broccoli florets, sliced
2 large boxes of vegetable stock
1 15 oz can of diced tomatoes
½ tbsp olive oil
Seasoned salt and black pepper to
    taste

1. To prepare, make sure that you have an Instant Pot.

2. On the setting, saute, add the olive oil, onions and celery. Cook until tender and turn the setting off.

3. Add all of the vegetables, stock, and can of diced tomatoes.

4. Set the instant pot to manual for 10 minutes.

_____

◇ **OPTIONAL:** Some people enjoy topping this soup with parmesan cheese or cilantro.

LETTUCE WRAP TACO

1 tbsp olive oil
1 lb ground turkey
1 cup salsa
1 4 oz can diced green chiles
1 tbsp taco seasoning
1 15 oz can corn kernels, drained
1 15 oz can black beans, drained
and rinsed
2 tbsp chopped fresh cilantro leaves
1 head butter lettuce
¼ cup shredded cheddar cheese,
optional
¼ cup reduced-fat sour cream,
optional

1. In a large skillet, cook the ground turkey on medium-high heat until fully cooked. Drain the excess fat.

2. To the browned turkey meat, add salsa, green chiles and taco seasoning until heated through, about 2-3 minutes.

3. Stir in corn, beans and cilantro until well combined; season with salt and pepper, to taste.

4. To serve, spoon several tablespoons of the turkey mixture into the center of a lettuce leaf, taco-style.

MOM'S TACOS

The aroma of tortillas frying in a pan full of Crisco brings us back to our roots. Our Mother used Crisco in so many of her recipes. These tacos are so amazing, full of grease and guilt. For health conscious folks, like ourselves, you can replace the Crisco (Is it still legal to sell anymore) with Extra virgin olive oil.

1 lb ground beef
2 tbsp Crisco
1 package of corn tortilla shells
½ medium red onion, diced
1 large tomato, diced
½ medium head of lettuce, shredded
1 cup shredded cheddar cheese
¾ tsp salt
1 tbsp chili powder
1 tsp ground cumin
½ tsp dried oregano
½ tsp garlic powder
¼ tsp black pepper
Optional Taco toppings: sour cream, taco sauce, or salsa.

1. In a large skillet, cook the ground beef until fully cooked.

2. To the meat, add the salt, pepper, chili powder, cumin, oregano, and garlic powder.

3. Reduce the heat to low and let it simmer.

4. In a separate frying pan, heat the Crisco over medium-high heat.

5. One at a time, warm each taco shell into the heated Crisco and allow each side to warm for roughly 1 minute. Heat the shell, but do not crisp it. The key is to remove the shell when it is warm but not fried.

6. Fill the warmed taco shells with a heaping of taco meat and top it with desired taco toppings: red onion, tomatoes, shredded lettuce, and more.

◊ **OPTIONAL:** Our Mother always had our taco shells super greasy and we loved it! If you are not a fan, set the taco shells on a paper towel to drain before eating.

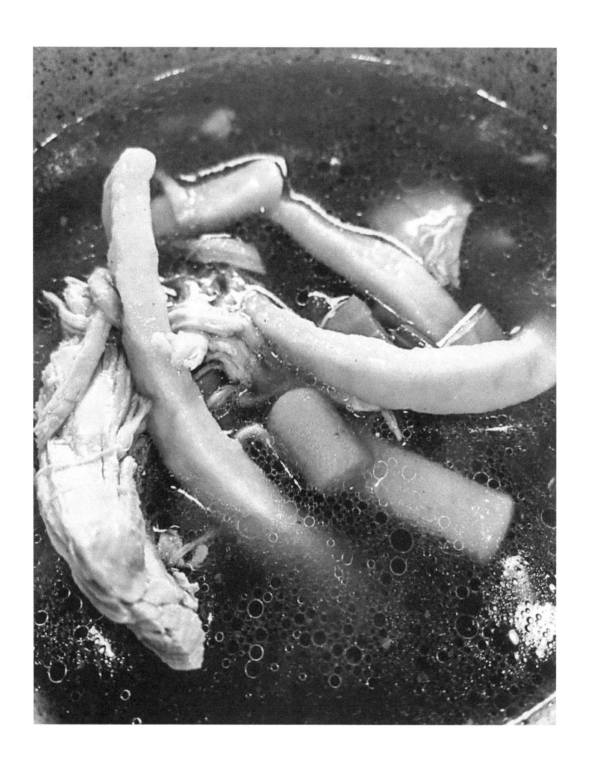

MOM'S CHICKEN NOODLE SOUP

This soup was a staple growing up. We wanted to honor our Mom's memory by sharing this recipe with all of you. Her secret ingredient was celery seeds and she never wanted us to share this secret. This soup is a perfect pair with our good health intention affirmations.

½ lb shredded rotisserie chicken
8 cups chicken broth
1 medium onion, diced
1 large carrot , sliced
2 celery stalks, sliced
12 ounces wide egg noodles
1 tsp thyme
½ tsp oregano
2 tbsp olive oil
Seasoned salt and black pepper to taste

1. In a large stockpot, heat the oil over medium

2. Add the carrots, onion, and celery & saute for about 7 minutes or until the veggies appear tender.

3. Add the chicken broth, thyme, oregano, salt, pepper.

4. Bring to a boil for 5 minutes.

5. Add the egg noodles and boil for 10 minutes or until the noodles are fully cooked.

6. After the noodles are done, turn the heat down to low-medium and add the chicken.

7. Let this simmer for 30 mins.

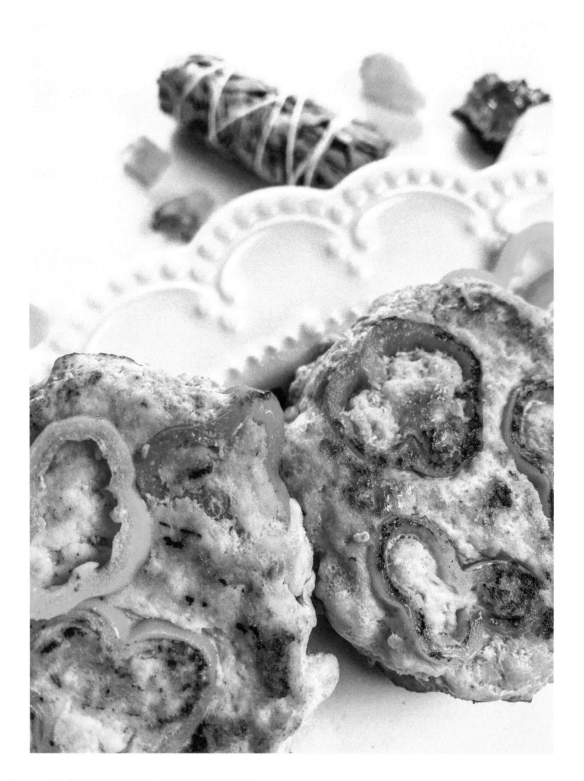

CHICKEN FAJITA BURGER PATTIES

1 lb ground chicken
½ medium onion, diced
5 miniature red bell peppers, sliced
1 packet fajita seasoning
2 tbsp olive oil

1. In a large skillet, heat the olive oil on medium-high heat.

2. Saute the onion and red bell peppers until tender.

3. Place the ground chicken into a large bowl.

4. Add the cooked veggies in the ground chicken and add the packet of fajita season.

5. Stir well until fully blended.

6. Heat 2 tbsp of olive oil in a large skillet.

7. Form the ground chicken into patties and place each patty into the heated skillet.

8. Cook the patties on each side for about 6 minutes until fully cooked.

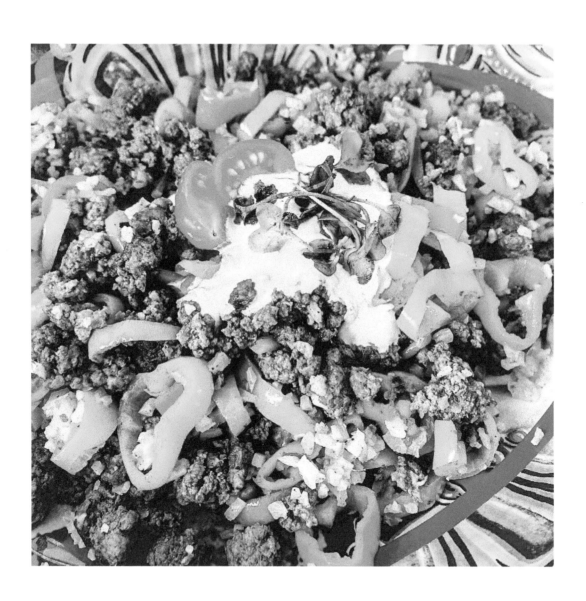

CAULIFLOWER TACO RICE

½ lb ground beef
½ medium onion, diced
½ medium red bell pepper, diced
1 packet taco seasoning, only use
   3 tbsp of the powder.
1 bag of cauliflower rice, frozen steam
   bags
2 tbsp olive oil
Seasoned salt and black pepper to
   taste

1. In a large skillet, heat the olive oil over medium-high heat.

2. Saute the onions and bell peppers in the skillet for about 7 minutes or until tender. Set aside.

3. Cook the ground beef until fully cooked and add the taco seasoning. Drain the extra fat.

4. Follow the directions on the bag of cauliflower rice and steam accordingly.

5. Add the cooked cauliflower rice to the cooked beef mixture. Add the cooked vegetables and stir.

6. Add more taco seasoning if you feel that this dish is not as spicy as you would like.

_____

◇ **NOTES:** This dish is great to add to a tortilla. Can be topped with cilantro and sour cream.

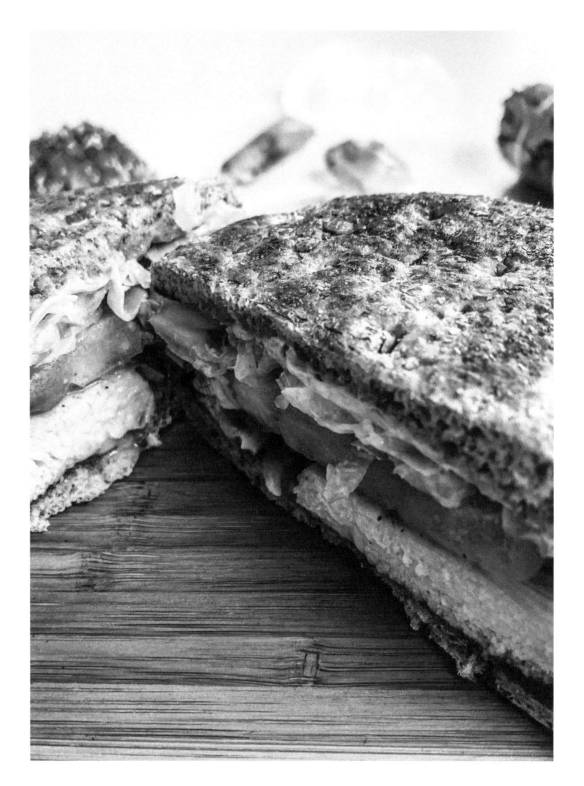

CHICKEN SANDWICH

1 package sandwich thins, wheat
4 chicken breasts, thinly sliced
½ medium red onion, sliced
1 bag of shredded lettuce
1 tomato, sliced
½ cup mayonnaise
1 tbsp butter, softened
2 tbsp olive oil
Seasoned salt and black pepper to
    taste

1. In a large skillet, heat the olive oil on medium-low heat.

2. Place the chicken breasts into the skillet and season with salt & pepper.

3. While the chicken is cooking, toast the sandwich things and butter each side.

4. Make sure the chicken breasts are cooked properly, roughly 7 minutes each side, with an internal temperature of 165 degrees.

5. Once the chicken is finished, start to assemble the sandwich by placing mayonnaise on each side of bread, tomatoes, lettuce, onion, and chicken breasts.

6. Serve while the chicken is warm.

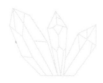

SUPER NACHO

1 lb ground beef
2 bags of tortilla chips
½ medium onion, diced
½ medium red bell pepper, diced
1 4 oz can of green chiles, drained
1 packet taco seasoning
1 15 oz can of refried beans
16 oz shredded cheese
3 roma tomatoes, chopped
Seasoned salt and black pepper to
taste

1. Preheat the oven to 400 degrees.

2. In a large skillet, brown the ground beef and onions for roughly 8 minutes or until fully cooked. Drain the excess fat.

3. Add the taco seasoning to the mean, stir evenly.

4. Add a large amount of tortilla chips to a baking sheet for the first row of nachos.

5. Spoon on refried beans, half on each pan. These are thick, so add a spoonful at a time all over the chips. (The spoonfuls will spread with the heat of the oven.)

6. Sprinkle half of the beef on top.

7. Sprinkle with half of the shredded cheese.

8. Repeat these same steps to create a second layer of nachos.

9. Bake at 400 degrees for 15 minutes.

10. Remove the nachos from the oven and add the bell peppers, and tomatoes.

◊ **OPTIONAL:** These nachos are amazing when served with sour cream, cilantro, or salsa. Add any additional toppings that you enjoy.

SHRIMP PESTO

1 lb large uncooked shrimp
1 tbsp unsalted butter
3 garlic cloves, minced
1 cup cherry tomatoes, halved
⅔ cup half and half
1 tbsp lemon juice
½ cup parmesan cheese, shredded
1 cup pesto sauce
Seasoned salt and black pepper to taste

1. In a large skillet, over medium-high heat, melt the butter.

2. Once the butter is melted, add the garlic. Cook for 2 minutes.

3. Add the half and half and bring it to a boil.

4. Reduce the heat and simmer.

5. Add the shrimp and cook for 1 minute.

6. Add the cherry tomatoes.

7. Cook until the shrimp are pink and done.

8. Stir in the lemon juice and the parmesan cheese.

9. Remove the heat and add in the pesto sauce, stir evenly.

10. Serve this over rice, pasta, or zucchini noodles.

KIELBASA STIR FRY

1 kielbasa, sliced
½ medium onion, diced
½ medium red bell pepper, diced
½ medium green bell pepper, diced
½ cup broccoli, broken into small pieces
½ cup cherry tomatoes, sliced
2 tbsp olive oil
Seasoned salt and black pepper to taste

1. In a large skillet, heat the olive oil over medium-high heat.

2. In the heated skillet, add the kielbasa and cook until done.

3. Remove the kielbasa and set aside.

4. Add all of the vegetables and cook them in the grease rendered from the kielbasa. Cook veggies until tender.

5. Once the vegetables are fully cooked, add the kielbasa and stir until fully reheated.

◊ **OPTIONAL:** This stir fry can be used over rice or cauliflower rice. Great to add over spinach also.

ZUCCHINI NOODLE PASTA

2 bags of frozen zucchini noodles
1 cup cherry tomatoes, halved
¼ cup lemon juice
2 tbsp unsalted butter
½ medium red bell pepper, diced
½ medium onion, diced
3 cloves garlic, minced
½ cup parmesan cheese, grated
Seasoned salt and black pepper to
　　taste

1. In a large skillet, heat the butter over medium heat.

2. Add the onions and red bell pepper into the heated butter and cook until tender.

3. Add the garlic and stir for 1 minute.

4. Add the cherry tomatoes and stir until full coated. Cook until softened.

5. Add the lemon juice and let simmer for 1 minute.

6. Follow the directions on the frozen zucchini noodles to prepare them.

7. Toss them into the mixture and coat evenly.

8. Add the parmesan cheese and fully coat.

9. Serve warm. Season with salt and pepper accordingly.

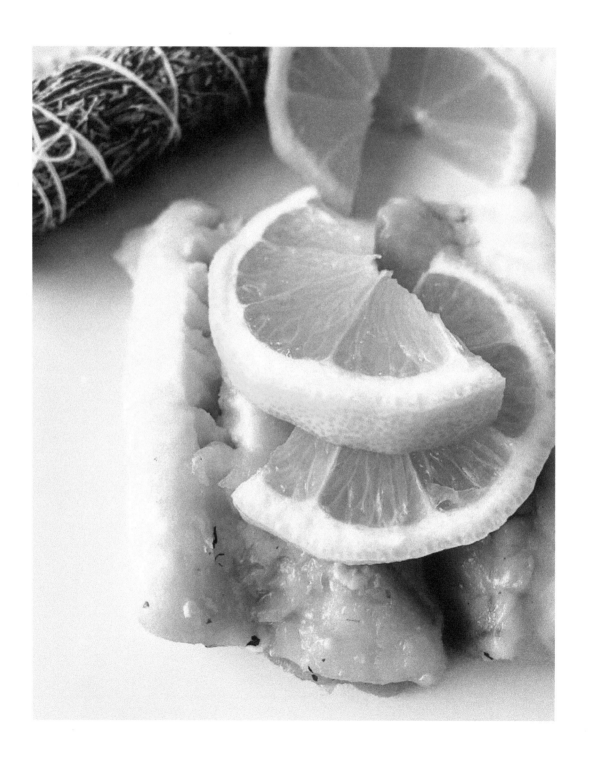

BAKED COD

1 lb cod fillets
1 tbsp lemon juice
½ lemon, sliced
1½ tbsp olive oil
Seasoned salt and black pepper to
    taste

1. Preheat the oven to 400 degrees.

2. In a baking tray, arrange the filets.

3. Drizzle the olive oil and lemon juice over the filets.

4. Season with salt and pepper.

5. Place the lemon slices on top of the filets.

6. Bake the cod in the oven for 10-12 minutes, depending on the thickness of the filets.

CAULIFLOWER RICE LEMON CHICKEN SOUP

1 large yellow onion, diced
2 tbsp of olive oil
2 stalks celery, diced
3 cloves garlic, minced
2 carrots, peeled and diced
1 teaspoon dried oregano
6 cups chicken stock
2 bay leaves
1 cup cauliflower rice
1½ cup rotisserie chicken
⅓ cup lemon juice
2 tablespoons chopped dill, fresh
2 tablespoons chopped parsley,
    fresh

1. In a large soup pot warm the olive oil on a medium heat.

2. Once warm, add the diced onion and sauté for about 3 minutes.

3. Add the celery and garlic and sauté another 2-3 minutes or until the onions and soft and translucent.

4. Add the carrots and oregano and stir for 1 minute.

5. Gently whisk in the chicken stock, bay leaves, and cauliflower rice.

6. Bring the soup to a boil and then reduce the temperature until it turns into a simmer.

7. Add the chicken and let simmer for 10 minutes.

8. Stir in the lemon juice and fresh herbs.

9. Season with salt and pepper to taste, and serve.

CHICKEN PARMESAN

4 boneless chicken breasts, halved
2 large eggs
1 cup panko bread crumbs
½ cup parmesan cheese, grated
2 tbsp flour
1 cup olive oil
¼ cup mozzarella cheese, sliced or cubed
Seasoned salt and black pepper to taste

½ cup marinara sauce see Dips & Sauces

1. Preheat the oven to 450 degrees.

2. In a large bowl, beat the eggs and set aside.

3. Mix the flour and parmesan cheese into a bowl and set aside.

4. Place the breadcrumbs in a bowl and set aside.

5. Coat each breast evenly by placing both sides into the flour mixture first, then the eggs, and coat in the breadcrumbs.

6. Set the breasts aside and let sit for 10 minutes.

7. Heat the oil in a large frying pan on medium-high heat until it is shimmering. Add each chicken breasts and fry on each side for 2 minutes.

8. In a large baking dish add the chicken breasts and top with marinara, and the mozzarella.

9. Bake at 450 degrees uncovered for 20 minutes.

◊ **OPTIONAL:** Topping this dish with fresh basil and grated parmesan is a great way to add color and flavor.

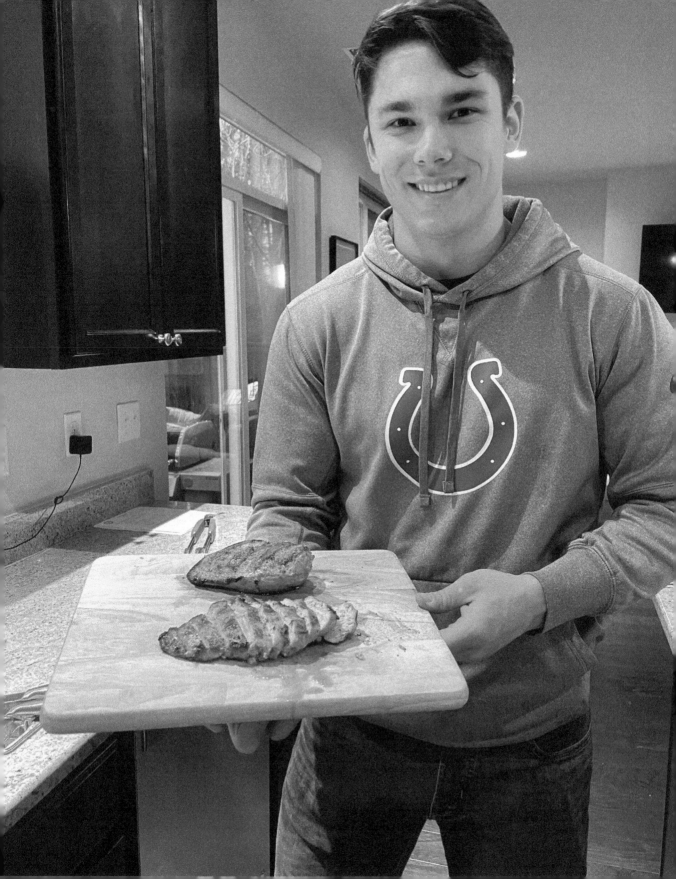

JOHN'S GRILLED CHICKEN

Christina here and I want to share a little fun fact with you. When John and I met, we were in the middle of a global pandemic. With restaurants closed, we had to spend our date nights at the house preparing our own meals. John's skills on the grill impressed me so much that it helped win over my heart.

I will never forget our fourth date. John had never grilled before but he decided to cook me dinner and he expressed the desire to use my grill. He told me he planned to wing it and warned me that dinner might not turn out. I trusted him and we prepared our dinner. John threw some seasonings together and started the grill. I put together a nice little Caesar salad. Dinner was ready and we were both nervous. Our bites were followed by moans and groans of how delicious we thought the chicken was. John's chicken is now often spoken about in our family and I request him to make it for me every week.

2 lbs boneless skinless chicken breasts
2 tbsp olive oil
1 ½ tsp salt
1 tsp garlic powder
1 tsp onion powder
1 tsp hickory seasoning
¼ tsp brown sugar
1 tsp black pepper

1. Preheat the grill on high heat.

2. IIn a large mixing bowl combine the chicken breast and olive oil, mix until the chicken breasts are completely covered in olive oil.

3. In a separate bowl, mix together all of the spices.

4. Add the mixed spices into the large bowl and fully coat the chicken breasts.

5. Set a timer for 10 minutes and set the chicken onto the grill.

6. After 10 minutes flip the chicken and grill the other side for another 10 minutes.

7. Allow the chicken breasts to rest for 5 to 10 minutes prior to slicing or serving.

TUNA MELT

2 6 oz cans of tuna, drained
2 dill pickles, finely chopped
8 slices of bread, sourdough or french
   preferred
8 slices of cheddar cheese
⅓ cup mayonnaise
2 tbsp unsalted butter, softened
½ lemon, for freshly squeezed juice
Seasoned salt and black pepper to
   taste

1. Preheat the oven to 400 degrees.

2. In a large bowl, mix together the tuna, mayonnaise, pickles, and lemon juice.

3. Butter each slice of bread on one side.

4. Add tuna mixture to the unbuttered side of your slice of bread, top with a slice of cheese, and sandwich together.

5. Face the buttered side up on a baking sheet.

6. Bake at 400 degrees for roughly 5 minutes or until the cheese is fully melted and tuna is warm.

CROCK POT BBQ RIBS

4 lbs baby back pork ribs
2 cups barbecue sauce
2 tbsp brown sugar
2 garlic cloves, minced
2 tsp worcheshire sauce
Seasoned salt and black pepper to
   taste

1. Spray a 6 quart crockpot with cooking spray and preheat it on low heat.

2. In a large mixing bowl, mix the barbeque sauce, brown sugar, garlic, worcheshire sauce, and salt and pepper.

3. Place the ribs into the crockpot.

4. Add the sauce and pour over the ribs.

5. Cover the crockpot and cook for 6-8 hours on low or until the ribs fall off of the bone.

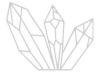

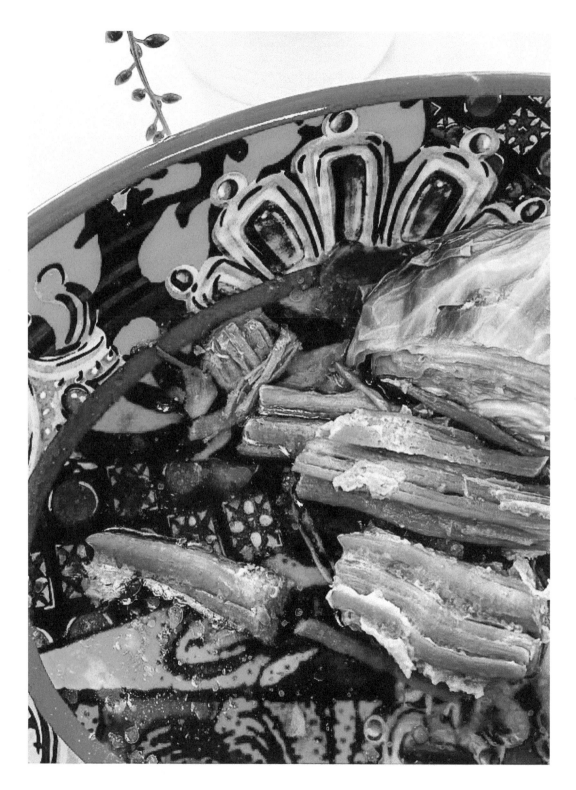

CROCKPOT CORN BEEF & CABBAGE

3 lbs of beef brisket with a spice
    packet included
1 large head of cabbage,
    quartered

1. Preheat a crock pot on medium heat.

2. Fill the crock pot with enough water to reach the max fill line after
   the beef brisket is added.

3. Put the spices from the packet into the water with the beef brisket.

4. Cover the lid and let the beef cook for 3 hours on medium heat.

5. After 5 hours place the cabbage into the crock pot for an
   additional 2-3 hours or until the meat is tender and the cabbage is
   cooked to your desired tenderness.

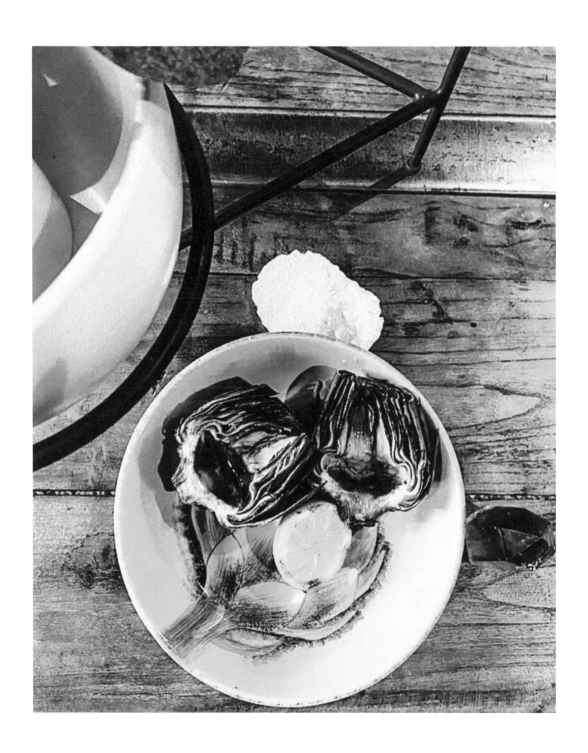

GRILLED ARTICHOKES

3 large artichokes
⅓ cup olive oil
1 lemon, quartered
Seasoned salt and black pepper to
   taste

1. Prepare a large pot of water. Boil the water.

2. Cut each artichoke in half.

3. Place the halved artichokes in water and boil for 20 minutes.

4. Prepare your grill on high heat.

5. Remove the artichokes from water and dry. Over the side opposite of the leaves with olive oil.

6. Grill the artichokes on the side of olive oil for 5-10 minutes.

7. Season with salt and fresh squeezed lemon juice.

◊ **OPTIONAL:** This dish is paired well with Garlic Aioli sauce. (See dips and sauces for the recipe)

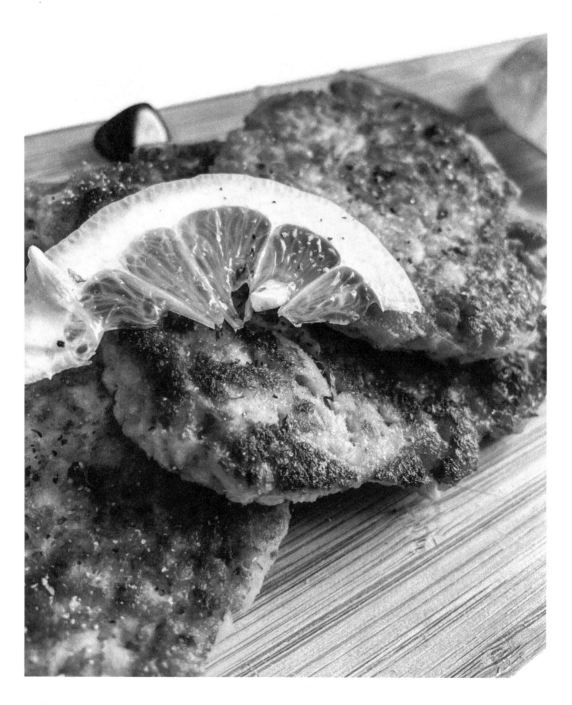

SALMON PATTY

1 14.75 ounce can salmon, drained of all but 2 tablespoons of the can liquid, flaked

1 slice of bread (crust removed), shredded

3 tablespoons green onion, chopped

1 garlic clove, minced

1 tbsp flour

1 large egg

½ tsp paprika

1 tsp lemon zest

2 tsps lemon juice

¼ tsp salt

3 tbsp olive oil

1. In a large bowl, mix salmon, bread, green onion, garlic, flour, egg, paprika, lemon zest, lemon juice, and salt.

2. In a large skillet heat the olive oil on medium-high heat.

3. Form the salmon mixture into 8 patties.

4. Cook the patties in the skillet until fully browned on each side, roughly 4 minutes per side.

◇ **OPTIONAL:** These patties are great when paired with fresh Tartar sauce. (See dips and sauces for the recipe.)

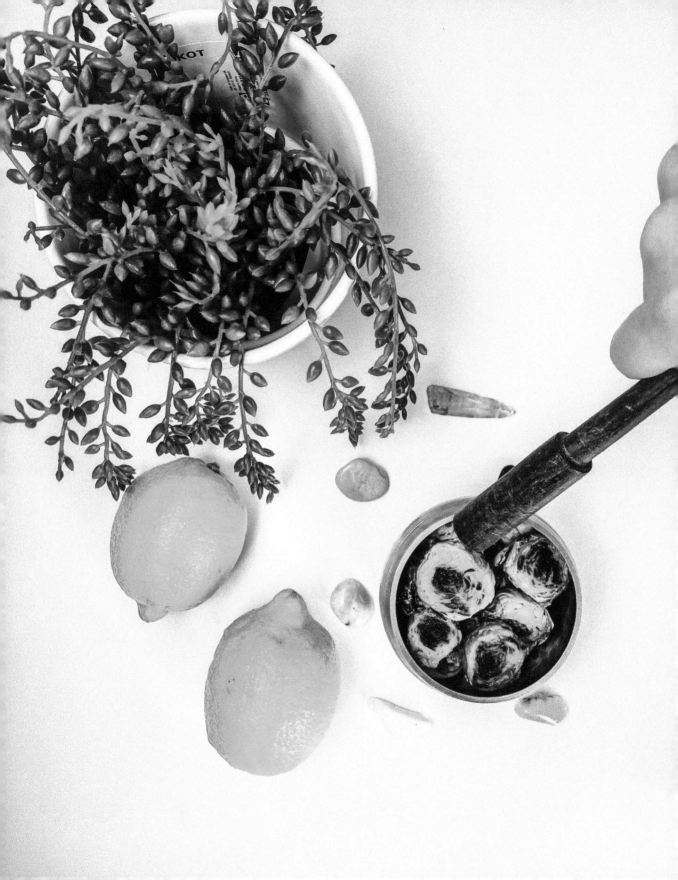

SIDES

BLT PASTA

Hello. Christina here. This is such a festive pasta salad to include at any potluck. My favorite time to make this dish is during the Fourth of July. This is one of those pasta sides that become an instant hit at anything I bring it to. My kids love it too, which is always an added bonus. I like to reiki charge this pasta dish with positive energy.

2 cups uncooked farfalle pasta
4 cups spinach, chopped
1½ cup tomatoes, chopped
4 slices bacon cooked to crispy, chopped
½ cup red onions, chopped

For the dressing:
¼ cup Ranch dressing
¼ cup sour cream
¼ cup mayonnaise
¼ tsp ground black pepper
1 Tbsp apple cider vinegar

1. Bring a large pot of water to a boil.

2. Cook pasta according to instructions on the box. Drain, rinse with cold water. Set aside.

3. In a small mixing bowl, combine all dressing ingredients and set aside.

4. In a large mixing bowl, add pasta, onions, bacon, tomatoes, and spinach.

5. Pour in the dressing and mix.

6. Can be eaten warm or cold.

MASHED SWEET POTATO

4 lbs sweet potatoes, peeled
⅓ cup butter, cut into 4 pieces
⅓ cup heavy cream
Seasoned salt and black pepper to
   taste

1. Bring a large pot of water to a boil.

2. Dice sweet potatoes into 2 inch cubes.

3. Add the potatoes to the boiling water and cook until tender,
   roughly 15 minutes.

4. Drain the potatoes and place in a large mixing bowl.

5. Add the butter to the potatoes and mash until butter is melted.

6. Add remaining ingredients and mash until the desired consistency
   is reached.

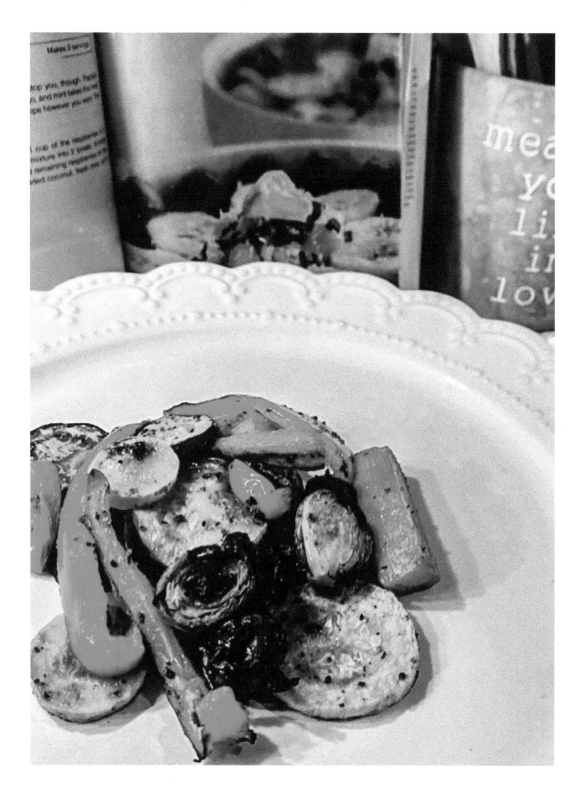

COCONUT ROASTED VEGGIES

1 sweet potato, cubed
1 garlic bulb, cloved
1 zucchini, diced
1 red bell pepper, quartered
1 carrot, sliced
2 tbsp coconut oil, melted
Seasoned salt and black pepper to
    taste

1. Preheat the oven to 400°F.

2. On a cookie sheet, drizzle half of the coconut oil

3. Add the cut and prepared vegetables, spreading them evenly on the cookie sheet.

4. Drizzle the remaining coconut oil on top of the vegetables.

5. Place in the oven on the middle rack and roast for 20-30 minutes or until the vegetables are brown and fully cooked.

6. Season with salt and pepper if preferred.

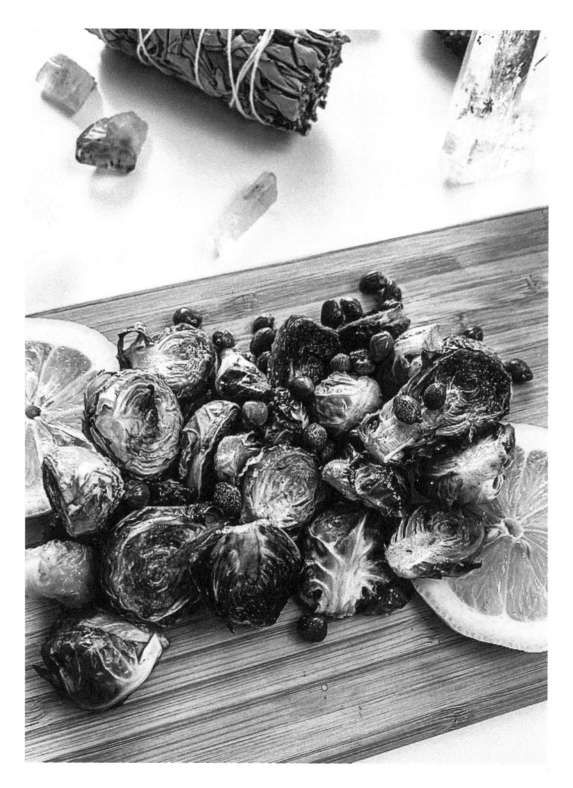

LEMON CAPER BRUSSEL SPROUTS

Hey, it's Jess here and this is one of my favorite side dishes to make. I enjoy pairing it with any meat dishes. It really adds an elegance to the dinner plate. If I could eat one food for the rest of my life, it would be Brussel sprouts. So it's natural for me to add some zaz to this vegetable. And since my favorite flavor is lemon this just all made sense.

2 lbs of brussels sprouts, halved
1 tbsp olive oil
1 tsp salt
2 tbsp capers
3 cloves of garlic, minced
½ lemon

1. Preheat the oven to 400 degrees.

2. In a medium size mixing bowl, combine the brussel sprouts, olive oil, salt, and minced garlic.

3. Mix well and then spread evenly onto a baking sheet.

4. Bake for 25-30 mins until they are crispy.

5. When finished baking, toss in a bowl with capers and freshly squeezed lemon juice from the lemon.

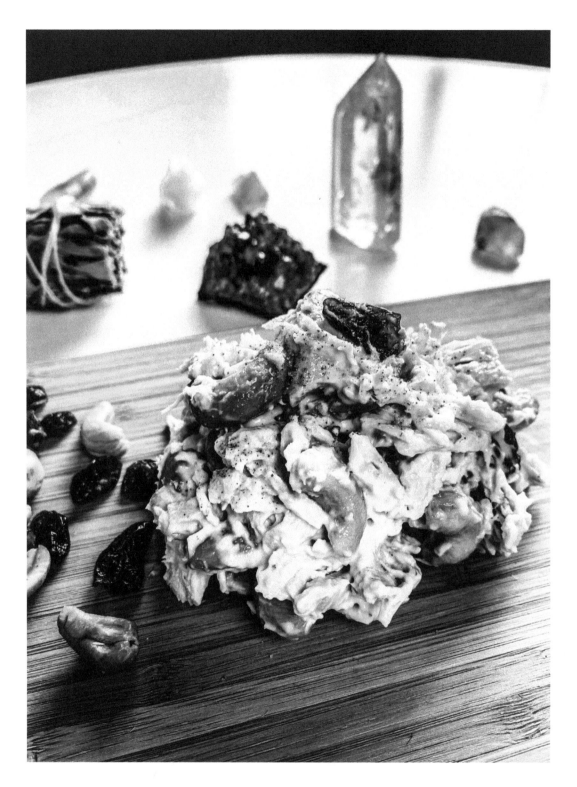

CHICKEN SALAD WITH CRANBERRIES

3 cooked chicken breasts, chopped
⅔ cup celery, chopped
⅓ cup red onion, chopped
½ cup dried cranberries
½ cup cashews
½ cup mayonnaise
1 tsp dijon mustard
Seasoned salt and black pepper to
    taste

1. In a large mixing bowl, combine the chicken, red onion, dried cranberries, cashews, and celery.

2. In a small mixing bowl, mix mayonnaise, mustard and salt & pepper, mix well.

3. Pour the mayonnaise mixture into the large bowl with chicken and until evenly coated.

4. Refrigerate for 1-2 hours before serving.

ROASTED CAULIFLOWER WITH FETA DIP

1 large cauliflower
2 tbsp of olive oil
Seasoned salt and black pepper to
  taste

For Feta Dip see Dips & Sauces

1. Preheat the oven to 400 degrees. Grease a baking sheet with olive oil.

2. Wash a large head of cauliflower and set aside.

3. Place the cauliflower onto the pre-greased baking sheet.

4. Drizzle the olive oil on the head of the cauliflower and place it face down, stem up, on the baking sheet.

5. Bake for 35-45 minutes.

SWEET POTATO FRIES

2 large sweet potatoes
2 tbsp of olive oil
Seasoned salt and black pepper to
taste

1. Preheat the oven to 400°F. Line a large cookie sheet with parchment paper.

2. Wash and cut the ends off of each sweet potato.

3. Cut the sweet potatoes into thin slices, roughly ¼ inches wide.

4. Place the cut potato slices into a large bowl and coat evenly with the olive oil and salt & pepper.

5. Spread the potato slices evenly on the cookie sheet.

6. Bake in the oven for 15 minutes, remove them and lightly flip and toss them.

7. Place back in the oven and bake for an additional 15 minutes.

8. Turn the oven off and let the potatoes continue to cook and crisp for another 30 minutes while the oven cools down.

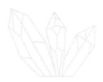

LUMPIA

1 package lumpia wrappers
¼ cup vegetable oil
5 garlic cloves, minced
2 lbs ground pork
2 tbsp soy sauce
2 large eggs, lightly beaten
6 oz cabbage, thinly sliced and
   minced
Seasoned black pepper to taste

1. In a large mixing bowl, combine the garlic, eggs, pork, soy sauce, dash of black pepper, and cabbage. Mix well.

2. Using a serrated knife, cut the square lumpia wrappers in half so that you have two stacks of rectangular wrappers. Place a damp paper towel over the wrappers to keep them from drying out as you work.

3. Place one of the rectangular wrappers vertically on your work surface with the short edge facing you. Place a heaping teaspoon of the filling on the wrapper about half an inch from the edge closest to you. Grasp the bottom edge of the wrapper and roll it up and over the filling, continuing to roll until 2 inches of wrapper remain.

4. Dip two fingers into a bowl of water, then moisten the last 2 inches of wrapper with your fingers. Finish rolling the lumpia, then rest it on its seam. Continue rolling with the rest of the filling and lumpia wrappers.

5. In a large skillet, heat vegetable oil on medium - high heat.

6. Place a few lumpia at a time into the skillet once the oil is fully heated. Cook each side roughly 5 minutes until golden brown.

LEMON PEPPER GREEN BEANS

1 lb fresh green beans, trimmed
2 tbsp butter
1 tsp lemon pepper seasoning
1 small lemon, halved
Seasoned salt and black pepper to
    taste

1. Bring a pot of water to a boil over high heat to prepare the green beans for blanching.

2. Add the fresh green beans to the boiling water and let blanch for 2 minutes.

3. While the green beans are blanching, melt the butter in a skillet on medium-low heat.

4. Remove the green beans and add them to the skillet.

5. Saute the green beans in the butter on medium-low heat.

6. Add the lemon pepper seasoning and continue to stir.

7. Saute the green beans for roughly 7 mins or until they are soft yet crispy in texture.

8. Squeeze one half of the lemon into the pan, stir.

9. Season with salt & pepper.

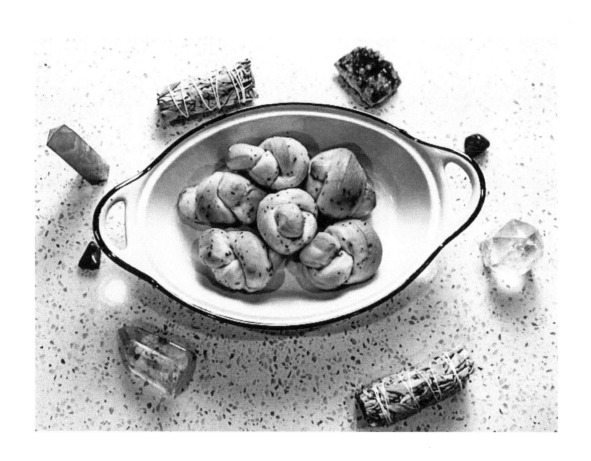

GARLIC KNOTS

1 lb of fresh pizza dough
¼ cup olive oil
5 garlic cloves
2 tbsp of fresh parsley
Seasoned salt and black pepper to
   taste

1. Preheat the oven to 400°F. Line a cookie sheet with parchment paper.

2. Roll out the pizza dough and cut it into ½ strips.

3. Roll each strip into a knot and place on the lined cookie sheet.

4. Place the garlic, olive oil, and parsley in a food processor or blender and blend until smooth.

5. Bake the pizza knots for 15-20 minutes until golden brown.

6. Add the garlic knots into a large bowl when finished baking and toss with the oil mixture. Season with salt and pepper to your liking.

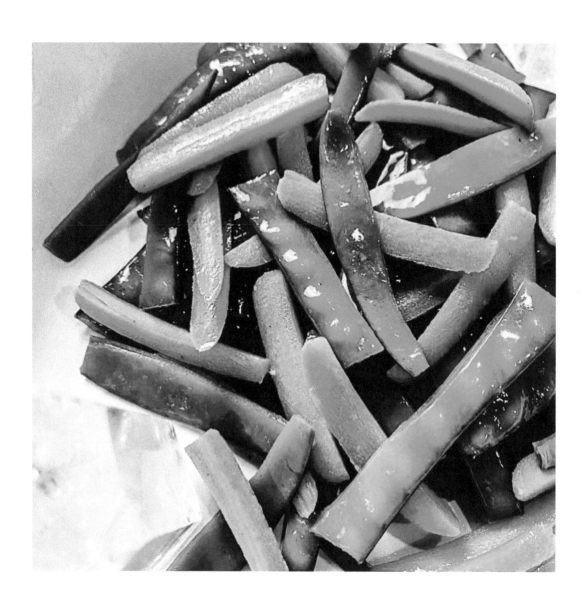

PEAS & CARROTS

4 large carrots, sliced
16 oz frozen peas
2 tbsp butter
1 fresh basil leaf, chopped
Seasoned salt and black pepper to
   taste

1. In a large skillet, melt the butter.

2. Add the carrots and peas and saute until tender.

3. Season with salt & pepper.

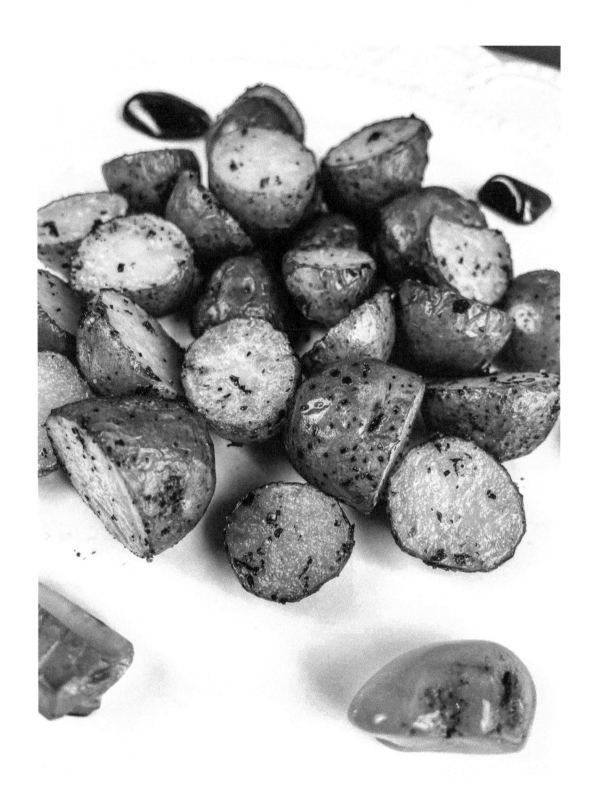

RANCH ROASTED POTATOES

2 lbs baby red potatoes, quartered
¼ cup olive oil
2 tsp Hidden Valley Ranch
   Seasoning
Seasoned salt and black pepper to
   taste

1. Preheat the oven to 450°F.

2. Place potatoes in a 1 gallon size Ziplock bag and add oil; seal bag. Toss to coat.

3. Add the ranch seasoning and toss to coat.

4. Place evenly on a baking sheet and bake for 30-35 minutes.

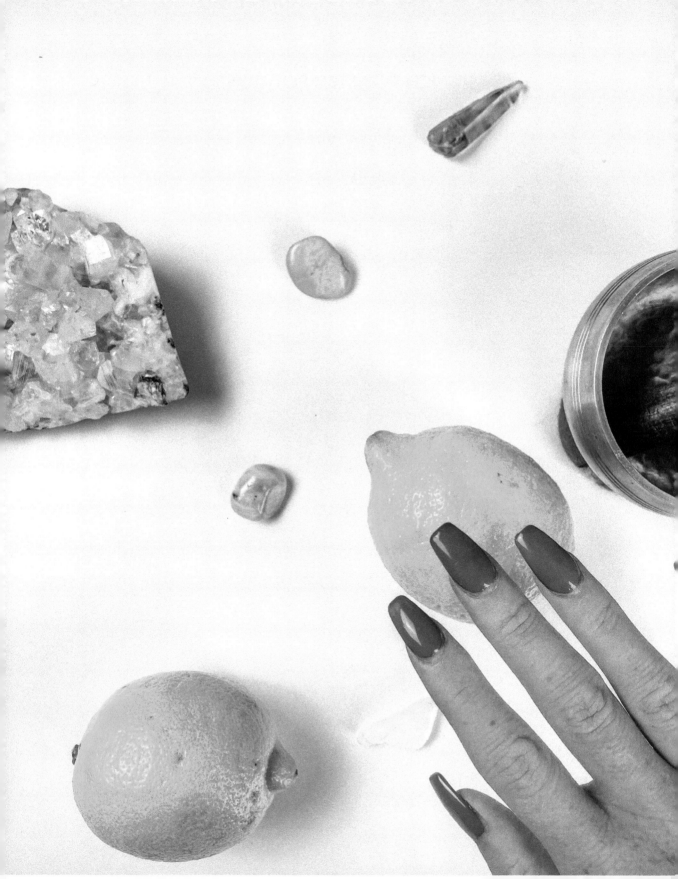

DIPS & SAUCES

LEMON GARLIC AIOLI

We are obsessed with artichokes and always use melted butter and garlic as our dipping sauce. It was good but we wanted to try something different. After a few trial and errors we found the perfect Aioli to dip our artichokes in. This pairs so well with them. It also can be used for so many other great recipes.

⅓ cup mayonnaise
⅓ cup low-fat Greek yogurt
1 tablespoon fresh lemon juice
1 teaspoon minced garlic
¼ teaspoon salt

1. Combine all ingredients in a bowl and stir thoroughly.

2. Add more garlic and lemon juice if needed for desired taste.

3. Refrigerate

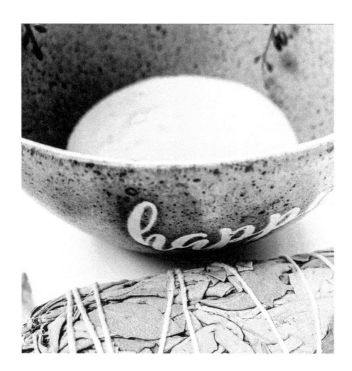

FETA DIP

1 cup feta
½ cup mayonnaise
½ cup Greek yogurt
1 garlic clove
Lemon zest
Seasoned salt and black pepper to
taste

1. Combine all ingredients into a food processor. Blend until smooth.

2. Add more salt and pepper if needed for desired taste.

3. Refrigerate and add a drizzle of olive oil over the feta dip when serving.

DILL SAUCE

1 can cream of mushroom
¼ cup of milk
2 tablespoons of fresh lemon
3 tablespoons fresh chopped dill
Seasoned salt and black pepper to
taste

1. Turn the stove on to medium heat

2. Combine all ingredients in a smaller pot and simmer for 5 minutes.

3. Stir until smooth and heated thoroughly.

4. Add more salt and pepper if needed for desired taste.

FRENCH ONION DIP

1 cup sour cream
1 tbsp dried chopped onion
1 tsp onion powder
½ tsp garlic powder
¼ tsp salt
1 tbsp dried parsley

1. Combine all ingredients in a bowl and stir thoroughly.

2. Refrigerate.

3. Serve cold with vegetables to dip or plain potato chips.

FRY SAUCE

Growing up we really didn't have much food in the house. My mom would often let us fend for what snacks to make. We always had potatoes so we would make homemade french fries all the time. One day we grabbed all our condiments out and made a fun sauce to dip our fries in. This is what we came up with and it's been in our family ever since. Simple yet so good.

¼ cup mayonnaise
¼ cup ketchup
Seasoned salt and black pepper to
  taste

1. Combine all ingredients in a bowl and stir thoroughly.

2. Add more salt and pepper if needed for desired taste.

3. Refrigerate

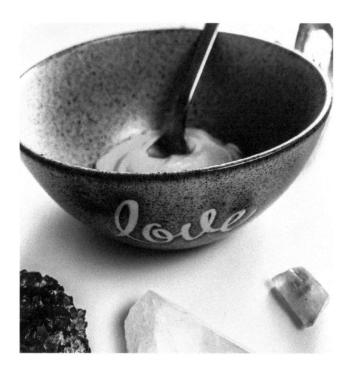

TARTAR SAUCE

1 cup mayonnaise
½ cup sweet pickle relish
1 tablespoon fresh lemon juice
Seasoned pepper

1. Combine all ingredients in a bowl and stir thoroughly.

2. Add more relish and lemon if needed for desired taste.

3. Refrigerate

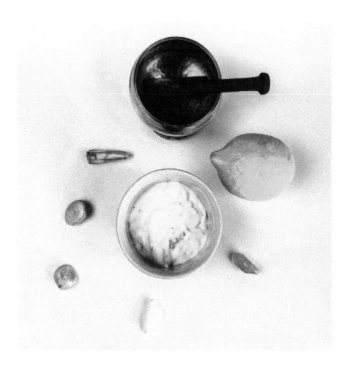

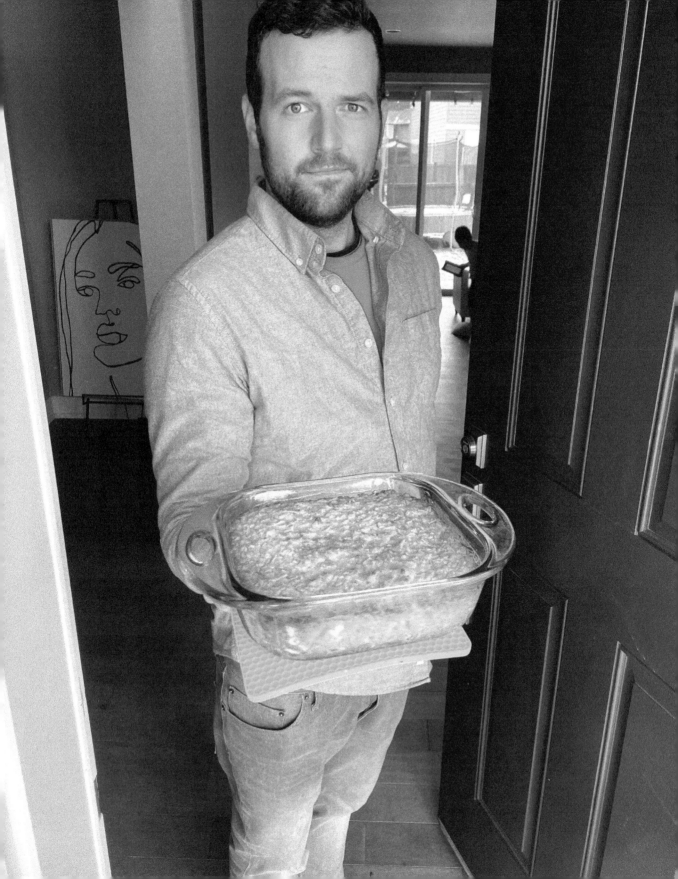

MIKE'S CRAB DIP

When Mike and Jessica were married, this crab dip was a part of every family gathering. It is passed down from his Mother, who made this dish on Easter when he was growing up. What was once a family tradition for him is now a family tradition for us. Even after a divorce, Mike is still a huge part of the family and we beg him to bring this crab dip to every event.

2 8 oz cream cheese, packaged
18 oz crab meat
1 cup mayonnaise
1 lemon, sliced

1. Preheat the oven to 325 degrees

2. Combine all ingredients in a bowl and stir thoroughly until the cream cheese is blended.

3. Place finished ingredients into a 9x9 oven safe dish.

4. Bake for 1 hour.

5. Place fresh lemon slices on top of dip as a garnish.

◊ OPTIONAL: This dip is paired really well with Pumpernickel bread.

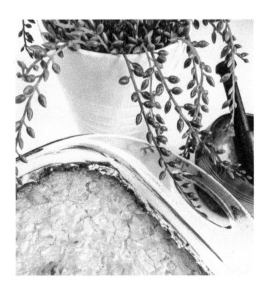

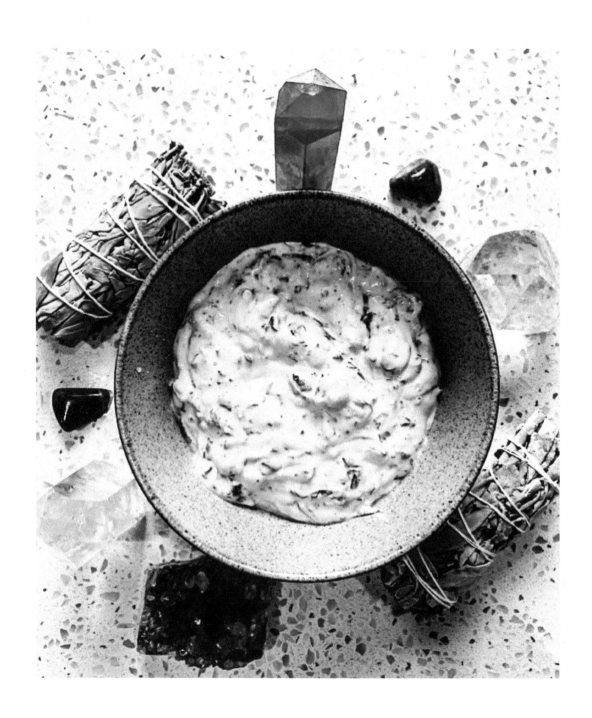

ARTICHOKE & SPINACH DIP

8 oz soften cream cheese
⅔ cup sour cream
⅓ cup mayonnaise
2 garlic cloves
1½ cups mozzarella cheese
½ cup shredded Parmesan cheese
10 oz frozen chopped spinach
14 oz chopped artichoke hearts
Seasoned salt and pepper

1. Preheat the oven to 375°F.

2. In a bowl, combine cream cheese, sour cream, mayonnaise, and garlic with a hand mixer until fluffy.

3. Stir in mozzarella and Parmesan cheese, spinach and artichokes.

4. Place in a 9x9 casserole dish and top with a bit more mozzarella cheese.

5. Bake until bubbly and brown on the top about 20-30 mins.

6. Remove from the oven and let cool down. Serve with bread or chips.

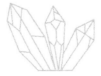

HONEY MUSTARD

½ cup mayonnaise
2 tablespoons yellow mustard
1 tablespoon dijon mustard
2 tablespoons honey

1. Combine all ingredients in a bowl and stir thoroughly.

2. Refrigerate and chill overnight.

MARINARA

1 large can (28 oz) whole peeled tomatoes
1 medium yellow onion, peeled and halved
2 garlic cloves

1. Combine all ingredients in a bowl and stir thoroughly.

2. Add more salt and pepper if needed for desired taste.

3. Refrigerate

ALFREDO SAUCE

½ cup butter, unsalted
1½ cups heavy whipping cream
2 garlic cloves, minced
½ tsp salt
½ tsp pepper
½ tsp Italian seasoning
2 cups parmesan, freshly grated

1. In a large skillet, heat the butter on medium-low heat.

2. Add the heavy whipping cream and stir.

3. Simmer over low heat for 2 minutes.

4. Whisk in the garlic, salt, pepper, and italian seasoning.

5. Stir in the parmesan cheese until fully melted.

6. Serve immediately.

HOLLANDAISE SAUCE

3 egg yolks
1 tsp dijon mustard
1 tablespoon fresh lemon juice
¼ tsp salt
½ cup butter, unsalted

1. In a mixing bowl, whisk together the egg yolks and melted butter.

2. Add the mixture into a heated skillet and simmer for 2 minutes.

3. Add the dijon mustard, fresh lemon juice, and salt.

4. Serve immediately while warm.

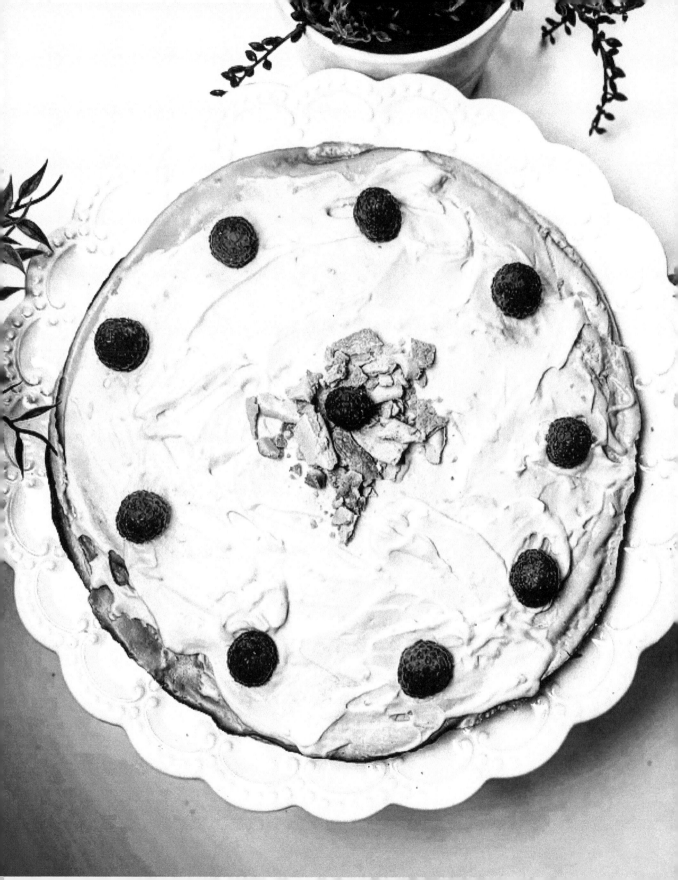

DESSERTS

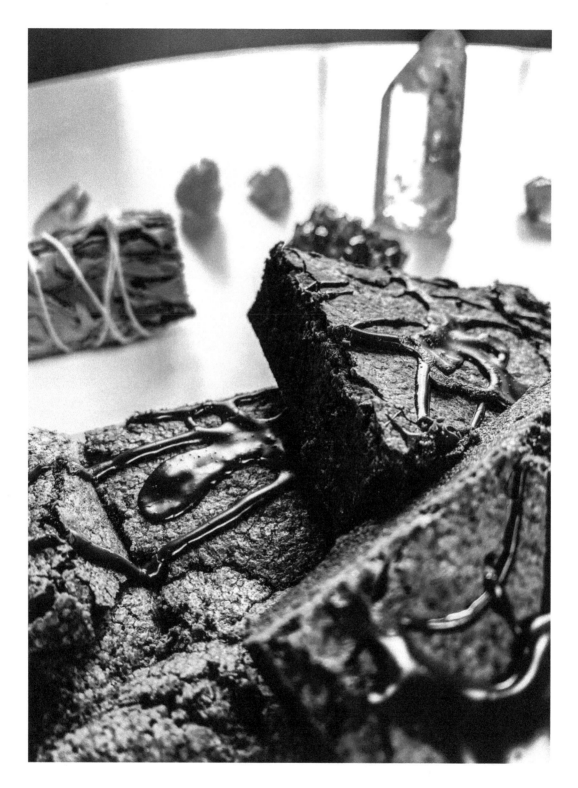

DOUBLE CHOCOLATE BROWNIES

1 cup white sugar
½ cup flour
⅓ cup cocoa powder
½ tsp salt
¼ tsp baking powder
½ cup chocolate chips
2 large eggs
1 tsp vanilla
½ cup canola oil (or vegetable oil)

1. Preheat the oven to 350°F. Grease an 8x8 inch baking pan.

2. In a large mixing bowl, combine sugar, flour, cocoa, salt and baking powder.

3. Stir in the chocolate chips and mix well.

4. Add the eggs, oil, and vanilla and stir until all is combined.

5. Spread the batter evenly into the baking sheet.

6. Bake for 25 minutes.

FRESH FRUITY MEDLEY

2 small apples, cubed
½ cup blueberries
½ cup raspberries
8 strawberries, halved
1 medium pineapple, peeled, cored,
   and cut into cubes
1 tbsp flax seeds
1 tbsp chia seeds

1. Mix all fruit in a large bowl.

2. Cover the fruit with flax seeds and chia seeds.

MOM'S PUMPKIN COOKIES

After our Mom passed away we both agreed that we often took many things for granted, her pumpkin cookies being one of those things. Each Thanksgiving, my Mom would prepare dozens of her cookies. They are so soft and chewy and we wish we would have savored every bite when she was alive. Now we prepare them using her recipe and we always make sure to reiki charge them with Gratitude.

2½ cups all purpose flour
1 tsp baking soda
1 tsp baking powder
1 tsp cinnamon
½ tsp nutmeg
½ tsp salt
1½ cups sugar
½ cup butter, softened
1 cup pumpkin puree
1 large egg
1 tsp vanilla
1 cup powdered sugar

1. Preheat the oven to 375°F. Spray a baking sheet with cooking spray.

2. In a large mixing bowl, combine flour, baking soda, baking powder, cinnamon, nutmeg, and salt.

3. In a separate bowl, mix with a hand mixer, beat in sugar, butter, pumpkin puree, egg, and vanilla.

4. Stir the dry and wet ingredients together.

5. Roll the dough into 1 inch balls and roll it in powdered sugar.

6. Place the dough on the baking sheet, 12 per sheet.

7. Bake for 11-13 minutes.

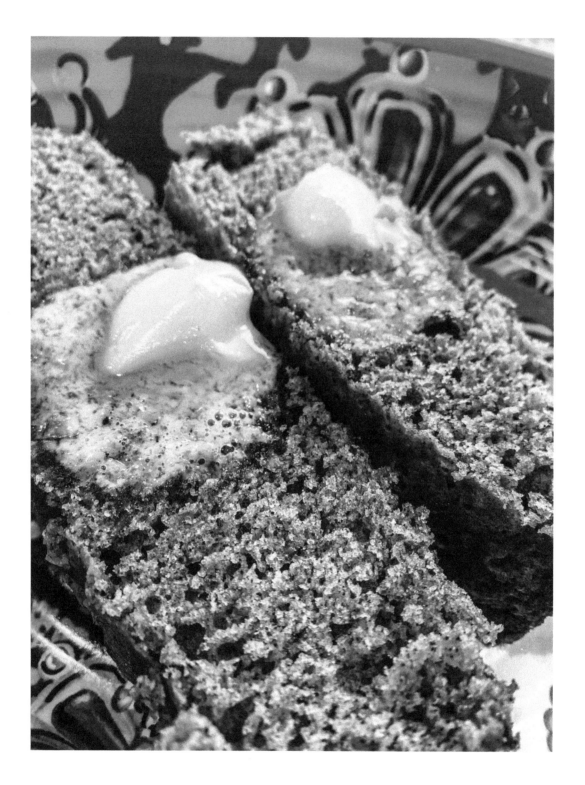

MOM'S ZUCCHINI BREAD

There was nothing more salutary than the smell of our Mom's fresh zucchini bread baking in the oven. Growing up we always had to smell the fresh aroma of cigarette smoke in the morning, therefore, to wake up to the smell of cinnamon was a breath of fresh air. We add humor because it was such a classic memory of ours.

3 large eggs
1 cup vegetable oil
2¼ cup sugar
2 large zucchini, peeled and shredded
3 tsp vanilla
3 cups flour
3 tsp cinnamon
1 tsp baking soda
1 tsp baking powder
1 tsp salt
½ tsp nutmeg

1. Preheat the oven to 350°F. Grease a baking loaf pan.

2. In a large mixing bowl, beat together the eggs and add the sugar gradually.

3. Add the oil, vanilla, and zucchini and mix well.

4. In a separate bowl, sift together the flour, cinnamon, baking soda, baking powder, salt, and nutmeg.

5. Mix the dry ingredients with the a mixture and stir evenly.

6. Pour into a greased loaf pan and bake for 1 hour.

◊ OPTIONAL: Growing up, our Mom always served this bread warm with extra salted butter. It would melt and add that extra delicious taste to this bread.

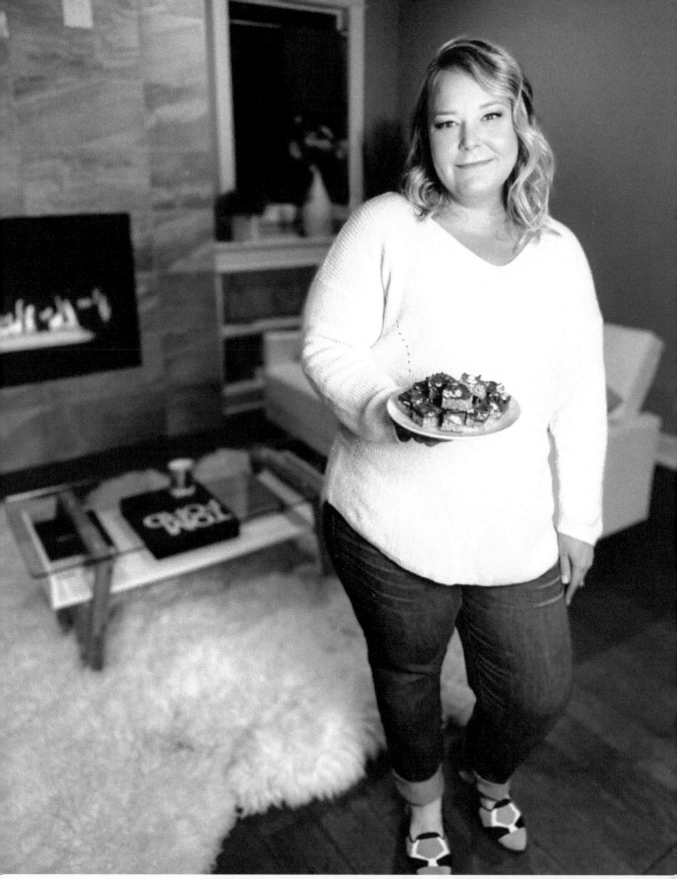

KAYLA'S BABY RUTH

Kayla has been our best friend since the fifth grade. She has always been a big part of our life. Going through all our ups and downs together. Her mother is also a big part of our lives. She is like a second mom to us. These are her family traditions at the holidays. To make batches of her Baby Ruth candies to pass out to family members. Every time we have a Christmas party Kayla always brings us a batch of freshly made Baby Ruth. It's one thing we always get to look forward to around the holidays. They have such a good flavor and really are a copycat to the original Baby Ruth candy bar. Not only do these candies look fabulous, they taste it as well!

Bottom Layer:
⅔ cups unsalted butter
¼ cup light corn syrup
¼ cup crunchy peanut butter
1 cup brown sugar
1 tsp vanilla
4 cups quick oats

Top Layer:
1 cup semi-sweet chocolate chips
1 cup butterscotch chips
⅔ cups creamy peanut butter
1 cup salted peanuts

1. Preheat the oven to 400°F. Prepare to first complete the bottom layer of this dessert.

2. In a large mixing bowl, add melted butter, corn syrup, brown sugar, crunchy peanut butter, vanilla and mix well.

3. Slowly stir in the quick oats.

4. Line a 9x13 baking sheet with parchment paper.

5. Spread the mixture into the pan and spread it out evenly.

6. Bake for 400 degrees for 10 minutes or until the edges are golden brown.

7. Set aside and prepare the top layer.

8. In a microwave safe dish, add the chocolate chips, butterscotch chips, and creamy peanut butter.

9. Microwave in 1 minute intervals and stir it until fully melted and smooth.

10. Mix in the peanuts and stir.

11. Pour the mixture over the bottom layer and refrigerate until it is hard and firm.

12. Cut into squares and enjoy.

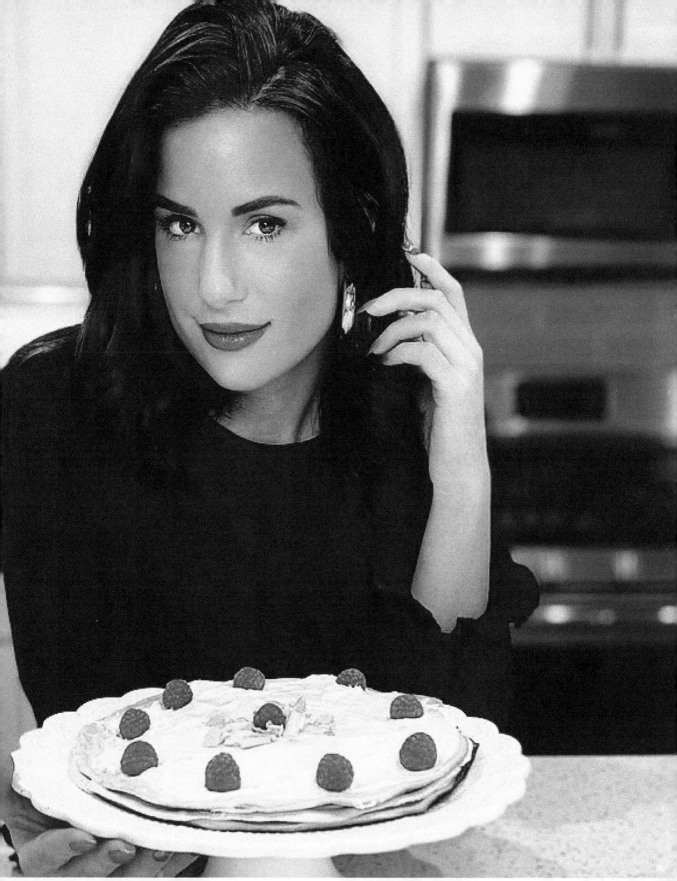

JESS'S LEMON TORTE

Hey, it's Jess! So here's a little fun fact about me. My all time favorite flavor is lemon. I am obsessed with anything and everything that has lemon flavor, from yogurt to lemonade. I tried this lemon torte at a Christmas party my boyfriend at the time invited me to. It was his Mother's tradition. She would make this torte every Christmas. I was instantly in love with these flavors. I couldn't stop thinking and talking about it after that night. I was able to have this dessert four times. That's how many years I dated this guy and was able to enjoy his family's tradition.

A couple years after being broken up I just couldn't stop obsessing over this amazing perfection. I was so sad that my taste buds may never get to experience such a heaven. So I ended up emailing his mother for the recipe and after a few changes I was able to perfect this dessert. I now use it as my Christmas tradition and make it once a year at my Christmas party. Now everyone asks me about it, and demands I make it. It is the hit of the party. I'm so glad I get to share it with you all.

4 large eggs, separated into egg whites only
½ cup sugar
¼ cup sugar
2 tsp sugar
½ tsp vanilla
4 large eggs, separated into egg yolks
3 tbsp lemon juice
2 tsp lemon zest
½ pint heavy whipping cream

1. Preheat the oven to 250°F.

2. Cover a baking sheet with parchment paper and draw three 8 inch circles.

3. In a large mixing bowl, beat the egg whites until stiff, adding the 2 tsp of sugar slowly, while continuing to beat consistently. Whip until stiff and the sugar is dissolved. Fold in the vanilla.

4. Spoon the meringue onto circles and level them out on the edges with a knife.

5. Bake at 250°F for 60 minutes.

6. In a large mixing bowl, beat the egg yolks with ½ cup of sugar until smooth. Add the lemon juice and zest.

7. Add this to a saucepan and boil the mixture while stirring constnatly until smooth and as thick as mayonnaise. Let this mixture cool.

8. In a separate bowl, whip heavy whipping cream until it holds stiff peaks. Gradually add ¼ cup sugar and vanilla.

9. Fold the lemon mixture into the whipped cream, using a spatula. Spread this between the meringue layers.

10. Refrigerate for 3 hours. Garnish the top with whipped cream and fresh raspberries.

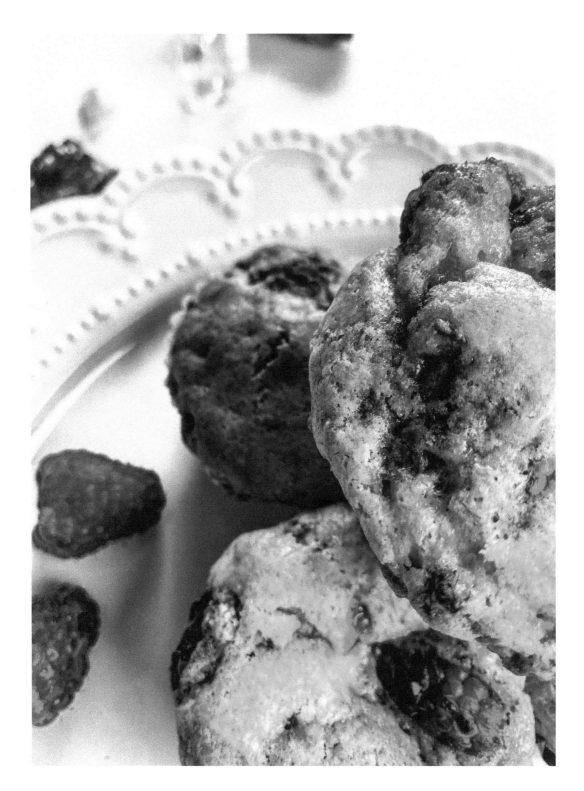

GLUTEN FREE RASPBERRY MUFFINS

1 package of Bob's Red Mill Gluten
   free muffin mix.
¼ cup fresh raspberries
½ cup vegetable oil
1 cup milk
1 large egg

1. Preheat the oven to 400°F. Grease a standard muffin pan or add liners.

2. In a large bowl, mix together the muffin mix, eggs, vegetable oil and milk. Stir until fully blended.

3. Add in the fresh raspberries, whole. Stir evenly.

4. Spoon the batter into each muffin pan.

5. Bake in the oven for the amount of time recommended on the muffin mix package.

6. In a large bowl, mix together the muffin mix, eggs, vegetable oil and milk. Stir until fully blended.

7. Add in the fresh raspberries, whole. Stir evenly.

8. Spoon the batter into each muffin pan.

9. Bake in the oven for the amount of time recommended on the muffin mix package.

MOM'S DONUTS

There were our favorite snacks that our mother made. She would spend all day making dozens of donuts. The one thing about our mom is when she would cook, she wouldn't just make one batch. It was an all day event in the kitchen. She always stored these donuts in an extra large mason jar that would be sealed airtight. The donuts are good for a few days and then start to harden, so eat them fast!

½ cup milk, warmed up
1 ½ tsp instant dry yeast
4 tbsp sugar
2½ cups flour
½ tsp salt
¼ tsp nutmeg
2 tbsp unsalted butter, softened
1 large egg
1 tsp vanilla
Sugar and cinnamon mixture for
   coating the donuts

1. Prepare your kitchen with a stand mixture, with a hook attachment.

2. In the mixer, add warm milk, sugar, and instant dry yeast. Let this mixture set for 5 minutes. It will start to look foamy.

3. After the mixture is foamy, add the egg and vanilla.

4. In a separate bowl, add the flour, salt, and nutmeg and mix together.

5. Add the dry ingredients to the wet ingredients and mix well with the mixer hook attachment.

6. After the ingredients are mixed thoroughly, by hand, kneed in the butter for 4 minutes until smooth and sticky. Place the dough into a greased bowl and cover with plastic wrap.

7. Let the dough set for 1 hour at room temperature. It should look doubled in size.

8. Dust a surface area with flour and roll the dough to a ¼ inch thickness. Using a donut cutter, cut the donut shapes and set them on a baking sheet covered with parchment paper.

9. Cover the tray of donuts with a clean kitchen sheet and set in the refrigerator to prove for 1 hour.

10. Heat Crisco oil to 350 degrees in a large pot or deep fryer.

11. Place the donuts into the oil for 30 seconds on each side before flipping. Continue to flip them until they reach a golden brown.

12. Remove the donuts from the oil and dip them immediately in the sugar/cinnamon mixture.

BANANA BREAD

1 Stick of unsalted butter
3 ripe bananas
2 large eggs
1 tsp vanilla
2 cups flour
1 cup sugar
1 tsp baking soda
½ tsp salt
½ tsp cinnamon

1. Preheat the oven to 350°F. Prepare a loaf pan by applying nonstick cooking spray.

2. In a microwave safe bowl, melt the stick of butter until it is softened.

3. Add the bananas to the same bowl and mash together with a fork.

4. Add the vanilla and egg and mix well.

5. In another large bowl, mix the flour, sugar, baking soda, salt, and cinnamon.

6. Add the banana mixture to the dry ingredients and mix it evenly.

7. Pour into the greased loaf pan and bake for 50 minutes.

NUTTER BUTTER MILKSHAKE

2 cups vanilla ice cream
¼ cup milk
2 tbsp creamy peanut butter
1 tbsp honey
5 nutter butter cookies
1 can of whipped cream topping
(Optional)

1. Prepare your kitchen by plugging in a blender.

2. Place the ice cream, milk, honey, and peanut butter in a blender and blend until smooth.

3. Place the nutter butter cookies into a ziplock bag and crush them. Keeping some pieces to be larger in size for texture.

4. Pour the cookies into the ice cream mixture and pulse blend only 3 times to just mix the cookies but not blending them too much.

5. Pour into a glass and top with whipped cream. Eating this with a spoon is recommended.

SMOOTHIE BOWL

1 cup frozen blueberries
1 small ripe banana
3 tbsp almond milk
1 scoop of protein powder of
   choice
1 tbsp shredded coconut
1 tbsp chia seeds
5 strawberries, sliced
3 tbsp almond butter, melted

1. Prepare the kitchen with a blender.

2. In a blender, add almond milk, banana, and protein powder.

3. Blend on high until smooth.

4. Add the frozen blueberries and blend until smooth.

5. Scoop the smoothie into a serving bowl

6. Top the smoothie with shredded coconut, chia seeds, strawberries.

7. Drizzle the smoothie bowl with the melted almond butter.

8. Eat right away or stick it in the freezer to enjoy later.

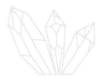

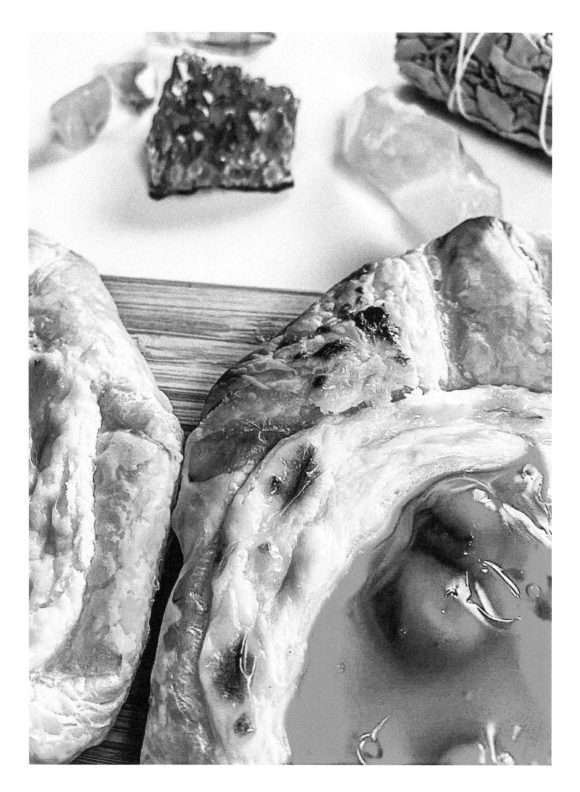

DANISH ROLL

1 can (8 oz) of crescent rolls,
   refrigerated.
3 tbsp powdered sugar
8 tsp of seedless raspberry jam
⅓ cup cream cheese

Glaze:
½ cup powdered sugar
3 tsp milk

1. Preheat the oven to 375°F. Prepare a cookie sheet.

2. Remove the dough from the can and do not separate it.

3. Using a serrated knife, cut the dough into 8 slices.

4. Place the rounds on the cookie sheet, 2 inches apart.

5. Press the center of each dough to create a ridge to place filling.

6. In a small bowl, mix cream cheese and 3 tbsp of powdered sugar.

7. Spoon each center of the dough with 2 tsp of cream cheese filling.

8. Top each cream cheese filling with 1 tsp of raspberry filling.

9. Bake for 12 - 14 minutes or until golden brown.

10. While the danish is baking, prepare the glaze.

11. In a small mixing bowl, mix the powdered sugar and milk. Add more milk if you desire a thinner consistency.

12. Drizzle the glaze over each roll once baked, and serve warm.

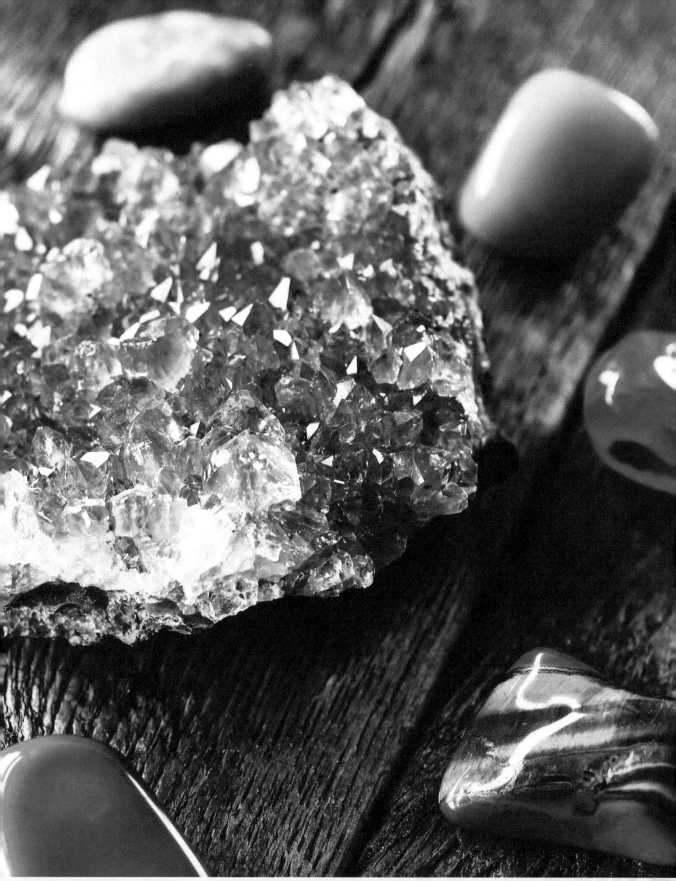

INDEX